Updates in HIV and AIDS: Part II

Editors

MICHAEL S. SAAG
HENRY MASUR

INFECTIOUS DISEASE CLINICS OF NORTH AMERICA

www.id.theclinics.com

Consulting Editor
HELEN W. BOUCHER

December 2014 • Volume 28 • Number 4

ELSEVIER

1600 John F. Kennedy Boulevard • Suite 1800 • Philadelphia, Pennsylvania, 19103-2899.

http://www.theclinics.com

INFECTIOUS DISEASE CLINICS OF NORTH AMERICA Volume 28, Number 4
December 2014 ISSN 0891–5520, ISBN-13: 978-0-323-32654-4

Editor: Jessica McCool
Developmental Editor: Donald Mumford

Infectious Disease Clinics of North America (ISSN 0891–5520) is published in March, June, September, and December by Elsevier Inc., 360 Park Avenue South, New York, NY 10010-1710. Periodicals postage paid at New York, NY and additional mailing offices. Subscription prices are $295.00 per year for US individuals, $510.00 per year for US institutions, $145.00 per year for US students, $350.00 per year for Canadian individuals, $638.00 per year for Canadian institutions, $420.00 per year for international individuals, $638.00 per year for international institutions, and $200.00 per year for Canadian and international students. To receive student rate, orders must be accompanied by name of affiliated institution, date of term, and the *signature* of program/ residency coordinator on institution letterhead. Orders will be billed at individual rate until proof of status is received. Foreign air speed delivery is included in all *Clinics* subscription prices. All prices are subject to change without notice. **POSTMASTER**: Send address changes to *Infectious Disease Clinics of North America,* Elsevier Health Sciences Division, Subcription Customer Service, 3251 Riverport Lane, Maryland Heights, MO 63043. **Customer Service: 1-800-654-2452 (US). From outside of the US and Canada, call 1-314-447-8871. Fax: 1-314-447-8029. E-mail: JournalsCustomerService-usa@elsevier.com (print support) or JournalsOnlineSupport-usa@elsevier.com (online support).**

Infectious Disease Clinics of North America is also published in Spanish by Editorial Inter-Médica, Junin 917, 1er A 1113, Buenos Aires, Argentina.

Reprints. For copies of 100 or more, of articles in this publication, please contact the Commercial Reprints Department, Elsevier Inc., 360 Park Avenue South, New York, New York 10010-1710. Tel. 212-633-3874, Fax: 212-633-3820, E-mail: reprints@elsevier.com.

Infectious Disease Clinics of North America is covered in *MEDLINE/PubMed (Index Medicus), Current Contents/ Clinical Medicine, Science Citation Alert, SCISEARCH,* and *Research Alert.*

Contributors

CONSULTING EDITOR

HELEN W. BOUCHER, MD, FACP, FIDSA
Director, Infectious Diseases Fellowship Program, Associate Professor of Medicine, Division of Geographic Medicine and Infectious Diseases, Tufts Medical Center, Boston, Massachusetts

EDITORS

MICHAEL S. SAAG, MD
Jim Straley Chair in AIDS Research, Professor, Division of Infectious Disease; Director, Center for AIDS Research, University of Alabama at Birmingham, Birmingham, Alabama

HENRY MASUR, MD
Chief, Critical Care Medicine Department, NIH, Bethesda, Maryland

AUTHORS

ANJU BANSAL, PhD
Assistant Professor, Division of Infectious Diseases, Department of Medicine, University of Alabama at Birmingham, Birmingham, Alabama

SUSAN E. BEEKMANN, RN, MPH
Department of Internal Medicine, The University of Iowa College of Medicine, Iowa City, Iowa

JOEL N. BLANKSON, MD, PhD
Department of Medicine, Johns Hopkins University School of Medicine, Baltimore, Maryland

AMANDA D. CASTEL, MD, MPH
Associate Professor, Department of Epidemiology and Biostatistics, Milken Institute School of Public Health, The George Washington University, Washington, DC

CATHERINE A. CHAPPELL, MD
Fellow in Family Planning and Infectious Disease, Department of Obstetrics, Gynecology and Reproductive Sciences, Magee-Womens Hospital of the University of Pittsburgh Medical Center, Pittsburgh, Pennsylvania

SUSAN E. COHN, MD, MPH
Professor of Medicine, Division of Infectious Diseases, Department of Medicine, Northwestern University Feinberg School of Medicine, Chicago, Illinois

ELLEN F. EATON, MD
Fellow, Division of Infectious Disease, University of Alabama, Birmingham, Birmingham, Alabama

JOEL E. GALLANT, MD, MPH
Professor, Division of Infectious Diseases, Department of Medicine, Johns Hopkins University School of Medicine, Baltimore, Maryland; Department of Specialty Services, Southwest CARE Center, Sante Fe, New Mexico

PAUL GOEPFERT, MD
Professor, Division of Infectious Diseases, Department of Medicine, University of Alabama at Birmingham, Birmingham, Alabama

ALAN E. GREENBERG, MD, MPH
Chair, Department of Epidemiology and Biostatistics, Milken Institute School of Public Health, The George Washington University, Washington, DC

DAVID K. HENDERSON, MD
Deputy Director for Clinical Care, Clinical Center, National Institutes of Health, Bethesda, Maryland

CRAIG J. HOESLEY, MD
Professor, Division of Infectious Disease, University of Alabama, Birmingham, Birmingham, Alabama

CHRISTOPHER J. HOFFMANN, MD, MPH
Assistant Professor, Division of Infectious Diseases, Department of Medicine, Johns Hopkins University School of Medicine, Baltimore, Maryland

MANYA MAGNUS, PhD, MPH
Associate Professor, Department of Epidemiology and Biostatistics, Milken Institute School of Public Health, The George Washington University, Washington, DC

JANET D. SILICIANO, PhD
Department of Medicine, Johns Hopkins University School of Medicine, Baltimore, Maryland

ROBERT F. SILICIANO, MD, PhD
Department of Medicine, Johns Hopkins University School of Medicine; Howard Hughes Medical Institute, Baltimore, Maryland

Contents

The reproductive health needs of all women of childbearing age should routinely address effective and appropriate contraception, safer sex practices, and elimination of alcohol, illicit drugs and tobacco should pregnancy occur. Combined antepartum, intrapartum, and infant antiretroviral (ARV) prophylaxis are recommended because ARV drugs reduce perinatal transmission by several mechanisms, including lowering maternal viral load and providing infant pre- and post-exposure prophylaxis. Scheduled cesarean delivery at 38 weeks with IV AZT decreases the risk of perinatal transmission if the HIV RNA is greater than 1000 copies/mL or if HIV levels are unknown near the time of delivery. Oral AZT should generally be given for at least 6 weeks to all infants perinatally exposed to HIV to reduce perinatal transmission of HIV.

Individual health benefits of antiretroviral therapy (ART) are becoming clearer. In resource-rich countries, side effects of current ART regimens are minimal. US guidelines recommend ART regardless of CD4 count or viral load. Maintaining an undetectable viral load with ART comes close to eliminating the risk of HIV transmission, leading the US guidelines to recommend universal ART to reduce HIV transmission. Achieving population-level control through treatment as prevention (TasP) may be feasible, but requires considerable investment of resources devoted to HIV testing, linkage to care, ART accessibility, and retention in care. Ongoing studies of TasP will provide insight into achieving meaningful ART coverage.

This article presents an overview of pre-exposure prophylaxis (PrEP) for human immunodeficiency virus (HIV) prevention. The authors describe the past animal and human research that has been conducted that informs our current understanding of PrEP; summarize ongoing research in the area, including describing new regimens and delivery mechanisms being studied for PrEP; and highlight key issues that must be addressed in order to implement and optimize the use of this HIV prevention tool.

> Condoms remain the most effective barrier against the sexual trans-mission of the human immunodeficiency virus (HIV). Male condoms have proven to be 80% to 90% effective, and female condoms have similar results. Poor adherence and improper use limit their effective-ness. In addition to condoms, microbicides are a promising barrier against HIV transmission. More than 50 candidate topical microbicide compounds have undergone preclinical or clinical testing in the last 10 years, but there are currently no US Food and Drug Administration (FDA)-approved compounds. Rectal microbicides are also being developed, as anal receptive sex is an effective mode of HIV transmission.

> Postexposure prophylaxis (PEP), which is designed to prevent human immunodeficiency virus (HIV) infection after an exposure, is one of several strategies for HIV prevention. PEP was first used after occupational HIV exposures in the late 1980s, with the Centers for Disease Control and Prevention issuing the first set of guidelines that included considerations regarding the use of antiretroviral agents for PEP after occupational HIV exposures in 1990. Use of PEP has been extended to nonoccupational exposures, including after sexual contact or injection-drug use. This article provides a rationale for PEP, assessment of the need for PEP, and details of its implementation.

> Although some success was achieved in recent years in HIV prevention, an effective vaccine remains the means with the most potential of curtail-ing HIV-1 infections worldwide. Despite multiple failed attempts, a recent HIV vaccine regimen demonstrated modest protection from infection. Although the protective efficacy in this trial was not sufficient to warrant licensure, it spurred renewed optimism in the field and has provided valuable insights for improving future vaccine designs. This review sum-marizes the pertinent details of vaccine development and discusses ways the field is moving forward to develop a vaccine to prevent HIV infection and disease progression.

> Remarkable advances have been made in the treatment of human immunodeficiency virus (HIV)-1 infection, but in the entire history of the epidemic, only 1 patient has been cured. Herein we review the fundamental mechanisms that render HIV-1 infection difficult to cure and then discuss recent clinical and experimental situations in which

some form of cure has been achieved. Finally, we consider approaches that are currently being taken to develop a general cure for HIV-1 infection.

INFECTIOUS DISEASE CLINICS
OF NORTH AMERICA

RELATED INTEREST

Clinics in Chest Medicine, June 2013 (Vol. 34, Issue 2)
HIV and Respiratory Disease
Kristina Crothers, *Editor*
Available at: http://www.chestmed.theclinics.com/

NOW AVAILABLE FOR YOUR iPhone and iPad

Preface

HIV/AIDS

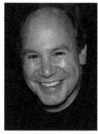 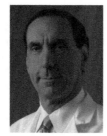

Michael S. Saag, MD   Henry Masur, MD
Editors

The last issue of the *Infectious Disease Clinics of North America* devoted specifically to HIV/AIDS was published in 1988. Edited by Merle Sande and Paul Volberding, that landmark issue provided a state-of the-art snapshot of the newly defined epidemic, its epidemiology, and the basic principles of treatment and care. Much has happened since then. In 2012, the number of persons living with HIV infection worldwide reached an all-time high of 35.3 million. The medical, social, and economic consequences of this global disaster have reached all continents, presenting society with a health-related challenge unlike any other.

Remarkably, the scientific community has investigated this epidemic and made dramatic discoveries with impressive speed. Considering that the first cases of the acquired immunodeficiency syndrome were reported in 1981, the ability of investigators to identify the causative agent in 1983, to develop a blood test in 1985, license the first active antiviral agent in 1987, and have durably lifesaving therapy a decade later is stunning. The partnership between clinicians, investigators, academic centers, government agencies, and the pharmaceutical industry has resulted in a life expectancy for HIV-infected patients with access to care that rivals that of their HIV-uninfected counterparts. In the 25 years since the publication of the last issue of *Infectious Disease Clinics of North America* on this topic, HIV has been transformed from a near-certain death sentence to a chronic, manageable condition.

Despite the remarkable scientific discoveries, the global community has not learned how to deliver effective therapy to the majority of infected patients in either the developing world or developed countries, such as the United States. Too many patients on all continents are not successfully engaged in care or provided treatment due to complex social, economic, and educational reasons. Thus, clinicians continue to be faced with patients presenting for care late in the course of infection, much as they did when HIV was first recognized in the 1980s, with a discrete constellation of opportunistic infections and neoplasms originally defined as "AIDS." Yet, modern clinicians also face a newer set of challenges by patients who are virologically well controlled on

Infect Dis Clin N Am 28 (2014) ix–x
http://dx.doi.org/10.1016/j.idc.2014.09.001
0891-5520/14/$ – see front matter © 2014 Published by Elsevier Inc.

antiretroviral therapy, but who suffer long-term metabolic, neoplastic, and infectious pathologies that limit the quality and duration of their survival.

These two issues of *Infectious Disease Clinics of North America* provide a comprehensive snapshot of the HIV/AIDS clinical field as it exists today. Like the last issue in 1988, these volumes focus on epidemiology, testing, and linkage to care, as well as antiretroviral therapy and therapy for the opportunistic processes. Some of these fields, such as the management of AIDS-related opportunistic infections, have changed a bit. However, other fields have changed much more dramatically, including what antiretroviral agents to start and when to start, metabolic and chronic viral co-morbidities, and strategies for the prevention of HIV infection, including pre-exposure and postexposure HIV prophylaxis, microbicides, and the concept of "treatment as prevention."

The authors of these articles are internationally recognized experts who summarize information that clinicians who care for HIV-infected persons should know in 2014 and beyond. Much has changed in the past 25 years in terms of manifestations, diagnosis, and therapy, but much more needs to change so that the number of infected persons globally shrinks, and so that long-term morbidity and mortality are reduced and ultimately eliminated.

Michael S. Saag, MD
Center for AIDS Research
University of Alabama at Birmingham
845 19th Street South/BBRB 256
Birmingham, AL 35294-2170, USA

Henry Masur, MD
Critical Care Medicine Department
NIH–Clinical Center 2C145
Bethesda, MD 20892, USA

E-mail addresses:
msaag@uab.edu (M.S. Saag)
hmasur@cc.nih.gov (H. Masur)

Prevention of Perinatal Transmission of Human Immunodeficiency Virus

Catherine A. Chappell, MD[a], Susan E. Cohn, MD, MPH[b],*

KEYWORDS

- Human immunodeficiency virus • Pregnancy • Antiretroviral medication
- Contraception • Perinatal transmission

KEY POINTS

- The reproductive health needs of all women of childbearing age should routinely address effective and appropriate contraception, safer sex practices, and elimination of alcohol, illicit drugs and tobacco should pregnancy occur.
- Combined antepartum, intrapartum, and infant antiretroviral (ARV) prophylaxis are recommended because ARV drugs reduce perinatal transmission by several mechanisms, including lowering maternal viral load and providing infant pre- and post-exposure prophylaxis.
- Scheduled cesarean delivery at 38 weeks with IV AZT decreases the risk of perinatal transmission if the HIV RNA is greater than 1000 copies/mL or if HIV levels are unknown near the time of delivery.
- Oral AZT should generally be given for at least 6 weeks to all infants perinatally exposed to HIV to reduce perinatal transmission of HIV.

PRECONCEPTION CARE

The purpose of preconception care (PCC) is to reduce unintended pregnancies, improve the health of women before conception, and encourage the use of safer conception strategies. The Centers for Disease Control and Prevention (CDC) and the American Congress of Obstetricians and Gynecologists (ACOG) recommend that PCC be performed as a part of routine medical care of all women and not something that occurs in a single visit, but rather a process that is integrated into routine health care visits to address the reproductive needs of women throughout their

Disclosures: The authors report no conflicts of interest.
[a] Department of Obstetrics, Gynecology and Reproductive Sciences, Magee-Womens Hospital of the University of Pittsburgh Medical Center, 300 Halket Street, Pittsburgh, PA 15213, USA;
[b] Division of Infectious Diseases, Department of Medicine, Northwestern University Feinberg School of Medicine, 645 North Michigan Avenue, Suite 900, Chicago, IL 60611, USA
* Corresponding author.
E-mail address: Susan-Cohn@northwestern.edu

Infect Dis Clin N Am 28 (2014) 529–547
http://dx.doi.org/10.1016/j.idc.2014.08.002
0891-5520/14/$ – see front matter © 2014 Elsevier Inc. All rights reserved.

id.theclinics.com

lifetime.[1-4] PCC is critical for all women, but can be particularly beneficial for women infected by the human immunodeficiency virus (HIV).

The benefits of PCC have been well described in reducing unwanted pregnancies and improving pregnancy outcomes.[2-4] HIV providers play an important primary role in the care of HIV-infected women, and are uniquely positioned to provide PCC and prevent unintended pregnancy. Prevention of unintended pregnancy in HIV-infected women and optimization of maternal health before a desired conception eliminates the risk of perinatal HIV transmission. However, discussions about reproductive desires frequently do not occur until after conception.[5-7]

Prevention of Undesired Pregnancies

With the introduction of highly active combination antiretroviral therapy (cART), live birth rates in the Women's Interagency HIV study (WIHS) cohort increased by 150% on comparing the pre-cART with the cART cohort.[8] Unfortunately, the most recent data from the United States indicate that nearly half (51%) of all pregnancies are unintended, with even higher rates associated with cohabitation, lower income, and lower education.[9] Studies in women living with HIV have reported an even higher rate of unintended pregnancy, possibly related to similar cultural and societal factors.[5,10-12]

Use of Contraception

HIV-infected women can potentially use all available contraceptive methods, including hormonal contraception and emergency contraception, as appropriate; thus, contraceptive counseling for HIV-infected women should be similar to that for uninfected women.[1] In general, counseling considerations of all contraceptive methods should include efficacy, safety, ease of use, cost, risks, potential noncontraceptive benefits, and protection against HIV and transmission of sexually transmitted infection (STI).[13] Contraceptive efficacy is one of the most important criteria women use when choosing a contraceptive method.[14-16] The World Health Organization (WHO) and the CDC have visual aids in discussing contraceptive options, and in general recommend that long active reversible contraceptive (LARC) methods, intrauterine devices (IUDs), and implants be promoted as first-tier contraceptive methods because of their superior contraceptive efficacy.[17,18] Both the copper IUD and the levonorgestrel IUD can be safely initiated or continued in women with HIV infection who are clinically doing well on combination antiretroviral therapy (cART), including those with AIDS.[19,20] The risk of spermicide use is generally contraindicated in HIV-infected women because of the increased risk of viral shedding and increased transmission caused by the disruption of the genital epithelium.[13]

Hormonal Contraception in Human Immunodeficiency Virus

Specific considerations for the use of systemic hormonal contraception in HIV-infected women include the potential risks of HIV disease progression, HIV transmission, and drug interactions with antiretroviral drugs (ARVs).[1] A recent systematic review of all studies evaluating the risk of HIV disease progression and hormonal contraception found only 1 of 11 studies showing an increased risk of declining $CD4^+$ count or death among women using hormonal contraceptives when compared with those using the copper IUD.[21] However, the study showing an increased risk of HIV disease progression with the use of a hormonal contraceptive had a very high rate of loss to follow-up and frequent method switching, and the intent-to-treat (ITT) analysis failed to show an association.[22]

There are also conflicting data on the role of hormonal contraceptives and the risk of HIV acquisition and transmission.[23] Three well-controlled studies have linked risk of HIV acquisition with progesterone-only contraceptives, most notably the injectable depot medroxyprogesterone acetate (DMPA).[24–26] Furthermore, HIV-infected women using DMPA for contraception had an increased risk of transmitting HIV to their male partners, and this risk was associated with increased genital HIV viral load.[26] These data are difficult to interpret considering potentially significant methodological concerns, such as difficulty accounting for behavioral confounders, presence of other STIs, and dependence on self-report for contraceptive use. Because of the uncertainty of the data and the significant benefit of hormonal contraceptives for maternal heath, the WHO has not recommend any restrictions on hormonal contraceptive use for women with HIV or at high risk of HIV. However, the WHO does call for further study of this potential association, and recommends increasing the contraceptive method mix and encouraging the consistent and correct use of condoms to prevent HIV transmission to noninfected sexual partners.[27]

Hormonal contraceptives that are primarily metabolized by the cytochrome P450 enzymes and specific ARVs, such as protease inhibitors (PIs) and nonnucleoside reverse transcriptase inhibitors (NNRTIs), can affect these metabolic pathways through induction or inhibition, resulting in decreased or increased levels of the components of hormonal contraceptives.[28,29] Drug interactions between ARVs and hormonal contraceptives are described in **Table 1**. Of note, these data are gathered from small pharmacokinetic studies, and few studies have shown that these hormonal changes have any impact on contraceptive efficacy.[1] In summary, efavirenz, nevirapine, and ritonavir-boosted PIs may increase metabolism of the progestin component of systemic hormonal contraceptives and decrease their contraceptive efficacy.[28,29] Thus, patients receiving cART should not rely on systemic hormonal contraception as their only method of contraception. Nucleoside reverse transcriptase inhibitors (NRTIs), CCR5 antagonists, and integrase inhibitors do not appear to have significant interactions with hormonal contraceptives and do not require alternatives or dose adjustment.[1] Because the hormonal levels achieved with DMPA are substantially higher than those required for contraception, any small reduction in hormonal level resulting from antiretroviral interactions is unlikely to reduce contraceptive effectiveness.[30]

Women Who Wish to Conceive or Are at Risk of Conception

PCC should take place when a woman desires pregnancy, she is uncertain about pregnancy, or she is not using contraception and is at risk for pregnancy.[13] Components of PCC are shown in **Box 1**. Reproductive decisions are shaped by personal, relationship, health, and financial factors that may make women reluctant to discuss these decisions.[31] Therefore, clinicians must initiate these conversations as part of routine care. All HIV-infected women contemplating pregnancy should be on a maximally suppressive antiretroviral regimen before conception to decrease the risk of perinatal transmission and transmission of HIV to an uninfected partner. In addition to HIV infection, overall health should be optimized and coordinated with other providers. Specifically, some chronic medical conditions, such as hypertension and diabetes, are associated with poor perinatal outcomes, and control of these disease processes decreases the likelihood of these adverse outcomes. Comorbid tobacco, alcohol, and substance abuse are commonly seen among HIV-infected women, and also are associated with poor perinatal outcomes. Couples should be counseled on safer sex strategies to prevent transmission to the HIV-uninfected male partner or transmission of other HIV strains with different antiretroviral resistance patterns from

Table 1
Drug interactions between selected antiretroviral agents and hormonal contraceptives

Antiretroviral Drug	Effect on Contraceptive Drug Levels	Clinical Recommendations for Combined Hormonal Methods and Progestin-Only Pills	Clinical Recommendations for Depo-Provera (DMPA)	Clinical Recommendations for Etonoregestrel Implant
Nonnucleoside Reverse Transcriptase Inhibitors (NNRTIs)				
Efavirenz (EFV)	Oral ethinyl estradiol/norgestimate: No effect on ethinyl estradiol concentrations ↓ Active metabolites of norgestimate (levonorgestrel AUC ↓83%; norelgestromin AUC ↓64%) ↓ Active metabolites of desogestrel (etonogestrel C_{24} ↓61%) Implant: 12.4% pregnancy rate with levonorgestrel implant Levonorgestrel (Emergency contraception) AUC ↓58%	Use alternative or additional contraceptive method	No addition contraceptive protection is needed	Use alternative or additional contraceptive method
Etravirine (ETR)	Ethinyl estradiol AUC ↑22% Norethindrone: no significant effect	No additional contraceptive protection is needed	No additional contraceptive protection is needed	No additional contraceptive protection is needed
Nevirapine (NVP)	Ethinyl estradiol AUC ↓20% Norethindrone AUC ↓19% DMPA: no significant change	Can consider an alternative method or reliable method of barrier contraception in addition to this method	No additional contraceptive method is needed	Can consider an alternative method or a reliable method of barrier contraception in addition to this method

Drug	Effect			
Rilpivirine (RPV)	Ethinyl estradiol AUC ↑14% Norethindrone: no significant change	No additional contraceptive protection is needed	No additional contraceptive protection is needed	No additional contraceptive protection is needed
Ritonavir (RTV)-Boosted Protease Inhibitors (PI)				
Atazanavir/ritonavir (ATV/r)	↓ Ethinyl estradiol AUC ↓19% ↑ Norgestimate ↑85%	Use alternative or additional contraceptive method	No additional contraceptive protection is needed	Can consider an alternative method or a reliable method of barrier contraception in addition to this method
Darunavir/ritonavir (DRV/r)	Ethinyl estradiol AUC ↓44% Norethindrone AUC ↓14%	Use alternative or additional contraceptive method	No additional contraceptive protection is needed	Can consider an alternative method or a reliable method of barrier contraception in addition to this method
Lopinavir/ritonavir (LPV/r)	Ethinyl estradiol AUC ↓42% Norethindrone AUC ↓17%	Use alternative or additional contraceptive method	No additional contraceptive protection is needed	Can consider an alternative method or a reliable method of barrier contraception in addition to this method
PI without RTV				
Atazanavir (ATV)	Ethinyl estradiol AUC ↑48% Norethindrone AUC ↑110%	No additional contraceptive protection is needed Oral contraceptive should contain ≤30 μg of ethinyl estradiol or use alternative method Oral contraceptive containing <25 μg ethinyl estradiol or progestins other than norethindrone or norgestimate have not been studied	No additional contraceptive protection is needed	No additional contraceptive protection is needed

(continued on next page)

Table 1
(continued)

Antiretroviral Drug	Effect on Contraceptive Drug Levels	Clinical Recommendations for Combined Hormonal Methods and Progestin-Only Pills	Clinical Recommendations for Depo-Provera (DMPA)	Clinical Recommendations for Etonoregestrel Implant
CCR5 Antagonist				
Maraviroc (MVC)	No significant effect on ethinyl estradiol or levonorgestrel	No additional contraceptive protection is needed	No additional contraceptive protection is needed	No additional contraceptive protection is needed
Integrase Inhibitors				
Raltegravir (RAL)	No significant effect	No additional contraceptive protection is needed	No additional contraceptive protection is needed	No additional contraceptive protection is needed
Dolutegravir (DTG)	No significant effect on norgestimate or ethinyl estradiol	No additional contraceptive protection is needed	No additional contraceptive protection is needed	No additional contraceptive protection is needed
Elvitegravir/ Cobicistat (EVG/COBI)	Ethinyl estradiol AUC ↓0.75 Norgestimate AUC ↑2.26	No additional contraceptive protection is needed	No additional contraceptive protection as needed	No additional contraceptive protection is needed

All recommendations are based on consensus expert opinion.
Abbreviations: AUC, area under the curve; C_{24}, 24-hour plasma concentration; C_{min}, minimum plasma concentration; DMPA, depot medroxyprogesterone acetate.
Data from Refs.[1,35,43]

Box 1
Component of preconception counseling for women living with human immunodeficiency virus (HIV)

- Discuss reproductive options; make appropriate referrals to experts in HIV and women's health when needed.
- Counsel on safe sex practices that prevent HIV transmission to sexual partners and acquisition of other sexually transmitted infections.
- Counsel on the elimination of alcohol, illicit drug use, and tobacco use.
- Counsel women contemplating pregnancy to take daily a multivitamin containing 400 μg folic acid to help prevent certain birth defects.
- Educate about risk factors for perinatal transmission and strategies to reduce these risks, including use of antivirals, mode of delivery, avoidance of breastfeeding, and infant postexposure prophylaxis.
- Optimize antiretroviral therapy regimen to maximally suppress viral load before attempting conception to decrease perinatal transmission and transmission to sexual partner.
- Adjust antiretroviral regimens to exclude efavirenz or other drugs with teratogenic potential.
- Optimize other maternal medical problems, such as diabetes and hypertension, before conception.
- Evaluate the need for appropriate prophylaxis or treatment of opportunistic infections, including safety, tolerability, and potential toxicity of specific agents when used in pregnancy.
- Administer any indicated vaccinations, such as influenza, pneumococcal, or hepatitis A or B vaccines.
- Offer all women who do not desire pregnancy effective and appropriate contraceptive methods to reduce the likelihood of unintended pregnancy.
- Offer emergency contraception as appropriate, including emergency contraceptive pills and the copper intrauterine device.

Data from Panel on Treatment of HIV-Infected Pregnant Women and Prevention of Perinatal Transmission. Recommendations for use of antiretroviral drugs in pregnant HIV-1-infected women for maternal health and interventions to reduce perinatal HIV transmission in the United States. Department of Health and Human Services. Available at: http://aidsinfo.nih.gov/contentfiles/lvguidelines/perinatalgl.pdf. Preconception Counseling and Care for HIV-Infected Women of Childbearing Age. Accessed March 29, 2014.

HIV-infected partners. Specifically, condom use should be encouraged at every act of intercourse. For couples desiring pregnancy, intravaginal insemination can be performed at home or in a physician's office.[1,13]

ANTENATAL CARE
Evaluation of Human Immunodeficiency Virus Infection in Pregnancy

Care of the HIV-infected woman during pregnancy requires close cooperation between prenatal care providers, HIV care providers, obstetric providers, pediatric providers, and other necessary services including mental health providers and substance treatment services. Initial evaluation of an HIV-infected pregnant woman should include assessment of HIV disease status (**Box 2**) in addition to recommendations regarding initiation of cART or alteration of a current cART regimen.[1] For women who initiate cART during pregnancy, providers should develop long-term plans

---

Box 2
Initial assessment HIV-infected women during pregnancy

- Review previous HIV history including previous opportunistic or HIV-related illnesses, previous HIV plasma viral loads, and CD4 counts.
- Document current plasma HIV RNA copy number and CD4 count.
- Assess the need for prophylaxis against opportunistic infections.
- Screen for hepatitis C virus and tuberculosis in addition to standard hepatitis B virus screening.
- Conduct baseline complete blood count and renal and liver function testing.
- Evaluate for immunization status of hepatitis A, hepatitis B, influenza, pneumococci, and Tdap.
- Test for HLA-B*5701 if abacavir use is anticipated.
- Take history of prior and current antiretroviral drug use, including adherence problems, side effects, and toxicities.
- Record results of prior and current HIV antiretroviral drug-resistance studies (will need a viral load of 500–1000 copies/mL for genotype testing).
- Assess psychosocial supportive care needs such as mental health services, substance abuse treatment, and smoking cessation.

Data from Panel on Treatment of HIV-Infected Pregnant Women and Prevention of Perinatal Transmission. Recommendations for use of antiretroviral drugs in pregnant HIV-1-infected women for maternal health and interventions to reduce perinatal HIV transmission in the United State. Department of Health and Human Services. Available at: http://aidsinfo.nih.gov/contentfiles/lvguidelines/perinatalgl.pdf. General Principles Regarding Use of Antiretroviral Drugs During Pregnancy. Accessed March 29, 2014.

---

regarding continuing cART postpartum, and considerations for continuing cART should be the same as for nonpregnant individuals. Furthermore, the impact of postpartum cART discontinuation is unclear, particularly with regard to women who have multiple pregnancies resulting in episodic receipt of ARVs.[32]

When to Start Antiretroviral Medications

Antiretroviral medications should be initiated for all HIV-infected pregnant women during pregnancy at the time of their visit documenting HIV infection plus pregnancy, and continued for those already at cART to prevent perinatal transmission and sexual transmission to an HIV-negative partner, and for the benefit of maternal health.[1] The use of any potent cART regimen that decreases the HIV RNA to undetectable levels in the plasma can significantly decrease the risk of perinatal transmission, the likelihood of cesarean section delivery to prevent perinatal transmission, and development of ARV-resistant HIV strains. In an analysis of perinatal transmission in 5151 HIV-infected women between 2000 and 2006 in the United Kingdom and Ireland, the overall mother-to-child transmission rate was 1.2%. A transmission rate of 0.8% was seen in women on cART for at least the last 14 days of pregnancy, regardless of the type of cART regimen or mode of delivery,[33] highlighting the primary importance of potent cART regimens in the prevention of perinatal transmission.

HIV can be transmitted from an HIV-infected woman to her child at any time during gestation, during delivery, and during the postpartum period through breastfeeding. Although most perinatal transmission of HIV occurs late in pregnancy or during delivery, early control of viral replication is important in preventing perinatal transmission earlier in the pregnancy.[34] However, teratogenic effects of drugs are of highest concern during the first trimester, and the risks of ARV exposure during this time are not fully known. The potential benefits of early sustained viral load suppression by starting cART in the first trimester must be balanced against the relatively unknown long-term outcome of first-trimester exposure of the fetus to ARVs, and the possibility of hyperemesis of pregnancy. Now that the DHHS Adult and Adolescent Guidelines recommend all patients with HIV be treated with cART regardless of CD4 cell counts and HIV RNA levels,[35] women should be encouraged to continue cART postpartum and lifelong. It is unclear whether women who receive short courses of cART during pregnancy and stop postpartum will be able to attain viral suppression during subsequent courses of cART.[1]

Antiretroviral Medications to Initiate in Women Who Are Antiretroviral Naïve

Combination cART regimens containing at least 3 drugs are recommended for all HIV-infected pregnant women to prevent perinatal transmission of HIV. Regimens should be individualized and selected based on the patient's comorbidities, convenience, side effects, drug interactions with other medications, ARV-resistance testing, pharmacokinetic changes in pregnancy, potential teratogenic effects, and overall experience of use in pregnancy.[1] The Panel on Treatment of HIV-Infected Pregnant Woman and Prevention of Perinatal Transmission places all ARVs into categories for use in pregnancy based on available data[1]:

1. *Preferred:* Drugs or drug combinations are designated as preferred for use in pregnant women when clinical trial data in adults have demonstrated optimal efficacy and durability with acceptable toxicity and ease of use; pregnancy-specific pharmacokinetic data are available to guide dosing; and no evidence of teratogenic effects or established association with teratogenic or clinically significant adverse outcomes for mothers, fetuses, or newborns are present.
2. *Alternative:* Drugs or drug combinations are designated as alternatives for initial therapy in pregnant women when clinical trial data in adults show efficacy, but 1 or more of the following conditions apply: experience in pregnancy is limited; data are lacking on teratogenic effects on the fetus; or the drug or regimen is associated with dosing, formulation, administration, or interaction issues.
3. *Use in special circumstances:* Drug or drug combinations in this category can be considered for use when intolerance or resistance prohibits use of other drugs with fewer toxicity concerns or in women who have comorbidities or require concomitant medications that may limit drug choice, such as active tuberculosis requiring rifampin therapy.
4. *Not recommended:* Drugs and drug combinations listed in this category are not recommended for therapy in pregnant women because of inferior virologic response, potentially serious maternal or fetal safety concerns, or pharmacologic antagonism.
5. *Insufficient data to recommend:* The drugs and drug combinations in this category are approved for use in adults but lack pregnancy-specific pharmacokinetic or safety data, or such data are too limited to make a recommendation for use in pregnancy.[1]

cART regimens during pregnancy usually consist of 2 NRTIs and an NNRTI or PI, consistent with the recommendations for treatment of HIV in nonpregnant adults in addition to what is known about use of the drugs in pregnancy and risk of teratogenicity.[1] Preferred regimens are listed in **Table 2**. Studies of zidovudine (AZT) in the prevention of perinatal transmission suggest that an important mechanism of

Table 2
Recommended antiretroviral drugs for HIV-infected women who are antiretroviral naïve

Drug	Comments
Preferred Regimens: Regimens with clinical trial data in adults demonstrating optimal efficacy and durability with acceptable toxicity and ease of use, pharmacokinetic data available in pregnancy, and no evidence to date of teratogenic effects or established adverse outcomes for mother/fetus/newborn. To minimize the risk of resistance, a PI regimen is preferred for women who may stop ART during the postpartum period	
Preferred 2-NRTI backbone	
ABC/3TC	Available as FDC, can be administered once daily, but potential hypersensitivity reaction (HSR). ABC *should not be used* in patients who test positive for HLA-B*5701
TDF/FTC or 3TC	TDF/FTC available as FDC. Either TDF/FTC or TDF and 3TC can be administered once daily, but potential renal toxicity. Should be used with caution in patients with renal insufficiency
AZT/3TC	Available as FDC, but disadvantages are that it requires twice-daily administration, has higher potential hematologic toxicity even though most experience of NRTIs with use in pregnancy
PI regimens	
ATV/r + a preferred 2-NRTI backbone	Once-daily administration
LPV/r + a preferred 2-NRTI backbone	Twice-daily administration. Once-daily LPR/r is not recommended for use in pregnant women
NNRTI regimen	
EFV + a preferred 2-NRTI backbone *may be initiated after the first 8 wk of pregnancy*	Concern because of birth defects seen in primate study; risk in humans unclear. Postpartum contraception must be ensured. Preferred regimen in women requiring coadministration of drugs with significant interactions with PIs
Alternative Regimens: Regimens with clinical trial data demonstrating efficacy in adults, but 1 or more of the following apply: experience in pregnancy is limited, data are lacking or incomplete on teratogenicity, or regimen is associated with dosing, formulation, toxicity, or interaction issues	
PI regimens	
DRV/r + a preferred 2-NRTI backbone	Less experience with use in pregnancy than ATV/r and LPV/r
SQV/r + a preferred 2-NRTI backbone	Baseline ECG is recommended before initiation of SQV/r because of potential PR and QT prolongation; contraindicated with preexisting cardiac conduction system disease. Large pill burden
NNRTI regimen	
NVP + a preferred 2-NRTI backbone	NVP should be used with caution when initiating ART in women with CD4 count >250 cells/mm^3. Use NVP and ABC together with caution; both can cause HSRs within the first few weeks after initiation

Integrase inhibitor regimen

RAL + a preferred 2-NRTI backbone	Limited data on RAL use in pregnancy, but may be considered when drug interactions with PI regimens are a concern

Insufficient Data in Pregnancy to Recommend Routine Use in ARV-Naïve Women: Drugs that are approved for use in adults but lack adequate pregnancy-specific pharmacokinetic or safety data

EVG/COBI/TDF/FTC fixed drug combination	No data on use of EVG/COBI component in pregnancy
FPV/r	Limited data on use in pregnancy
MVC	MVC requires tropism testing before use. Few case reports of use in pregnancy
RPV	RPV not recommended with pretreatment HIV RNA >100,000 copies/mL or CD4 count <200 cells/mm^3. Do not use with proton-pump inhibitor. Limited data on use in pregnancy
DTG	Limited data on use in pregnancy

Not Recommended: Drugs whose use is not recommended because of toxicity, lower rate of viral suppression, or because no recommendation in naïve populations

ABC/3TC/AZT	Not recommended owing to inferior virologic efficacy
d4T	Not recommended because of toxicity
ddI	Not recommended because of toxicity
IDV/r	Concerns regarding kidney stones, hyperbilirubinemia
NFV	Lower rate of viral suppression with NFV compared with LPV/r or EFV in adult trials
RTV	Ritonavir as a single PI is not recommended because of inferior efficacy and increased toxicity
ETR	Not recommended in naïve populations
T20	Not recommended in naïve populations
TPV	Not recommended in naïve populations

Abbreviations: 3TC, lamivudine; ABC, abacavir; ART, antiretroviral therapy; ATV/r, atazanavir/ritonavir; AZT, zidovudine; DRV/r, darunavir/ritonavir; DTG, dolutegravir; ECG, electrocardiogram; EFV, efavirenz; ETR, etravirine; EVG/COBI, elvitegravir/cobicistat; FDC, fixed drug combination; FTC, emtricitabine; HSR, hypersensitivity reaction; IDV/r, indinavir/ritonavir; LPV/r, lopinavir/ritonavir; MVC, maraviroc; NNRTI, nonnucleoside reverse transcriptase inhibitor; NRTI, nucleoside reverse transcriptase inhibitor; NVP, nevirapine; PI, protease inhibitor; RAL, raltegravir; RPV, rilpivirine; RTV, ritonavir; T20, enfurvirtide; TDF, tenofovir disoproxil fumarate; TPV, tipranavir.

infant preexposure prophylaxis is transplacental drug passage. Thus, when selecting cART regimen for pregnant women, at least 1 NRTI agent with high placental transfer should be included (AZT, lamivudine, emtricitabine, tenofovir, or abacavir). Alternative regimens can be used in women who are intolerant of or have developed toxicity to the preferred regimen, or have noted resistance. Pregnancy-specific information on all available ARVs can be found at: http://www.aidsinfo.nih.gov/contentfiles/lvguidelines/perinatalgl.pdf (Table 7, pp. 62–76; accessed March 30, 2014).[1] Specific situations when alternative regimens should be considered are listed in **Table 2**.

ARV-resistance testing should be performed before starting the regimen if the HIV RNA viral load is higher than 500 to 1000 copies/mL. However, given that early sustained viral load suppression is associated with a decreased likelihood for perinatal transmission, cART regimens should be initiated promptly even before receiving the resistance-testing results, especially if HIV is diagnosed in the second or third trimesters of pregnancy. In the cases where ARV-resistance testing is unavailable, consideration should be given to staring a PI-based cART regimen, owing to the higher barrier for resistance of the PIs in comparison with the NNRTIs.[1]

A noted difference between the preferred cART regimens for adults and the preferred cART regimens for pregnant women is the lack of integrase inhibitor–based regimens for pregnant women. Data on use of the integrase inhibitor raltegravir during pregnancy are currently limited, though increasing. Raltegravir may be considered for use in late pregnancy for women with high HIV RNA viral loads because of its ability to rapidly suppress viremia.[36] However, the efficacy and safety of this approach has not been evaluated, and thus cannot be recommended.[1]

Antiretroviral Medications to Start in Women Who Are Antiretroviral Experienced

In general, HIV-infected women who are currently receiving cART should be continued on that cART regimen, assuming that it has been well tolerated and is effectively suppressing viral replication to undetectable levels. Discontinuation or switching of cART could lead to HIV viremia and an increased risk of perinatal HIV transmission. The potential concerns for teratogenic effects of ARVs in the first trimester are outweighed by the benefits of continuation of the cART regimen for maternal health and prevention of perinatal transmission, thus continuation of cART is recommended.[1]

There are specific concerns for the use of efavirenz in the first trimester because of a potential association with neural tube defects, based on preclinical primate data and retrospective case reports. A recent meta-analysis did not find an increased relative risk (RR) of overall birth defects in infants born to women receiving efavirenz-based versus non-efavirenz–based regimens (RR 0.85, 95% confidence interval [CI] 0.6–1.2), and identified 1 neural tube defect, resulting in an incidence of 0.07% (95% CI 0.002%–0.39%).[37] The available data suggest that first-trimester exposure is not associated with a large (ie, 10-fold or more) increase in risk of neural tube defects, although a small increase in risk of a rare outcome cannot be ruled out. The risk of neural tube defects is restricted to the first 5 to 6 weeks of pregnancy (the neural tube closes at 36–39 days after last menstrual period); pregnancy is rarely recognized before 4 to 6 weeks of pregnancy, and unnecessary changes of ARVs in pregnancy may be associated with loss of viral control and, thus, increased risk of transmission to the infant. Therefore, HIV-infected pregnant women who are well controlled on efavirenz-based cART should be continued on this regimen through the duration of pregnancy.[1]

In addition, there is concern that some women with previous time-limited use of ARVs during previous pregnancies may develop genotypic resistance to 1 or more components of the initial ARV regimen, thus potentially limiting the efficacy of standard regimens (ie, those containing the dual NRTI backbone of AZT and lamivudine [3TC]).

Given the lack of substantive data, it is reasonable to make preliminary decisions about cART regimens based on results of previous resistance testing. Careful monitoring of virologic response to the chosen cART regimen is important, and adjustments to therapy should be guided by repeat resistance testing in consultation with a clinician experienced in HIV treatment.[1]

If an HIV-infected pregnant woman has detectable HIV viremia (ie, >500–1000 copies/mL) while on cART, adherence counseling and HIV-resistance testing should be performed. She should have a follow-up viral load test and, if HIV is still detectable, her cART should be adjusted based on her HIV-resistance testing, as with nonpregnant patients.[1]

Monitoring the Woman and the Fetus After Initiation of Antiretroviral Therapy

CD4 counts should be monitored in HIV-infected pregnant women at the initial visit and at least every 3 to 6 months during pregnancy, similarly to recommendations for nonpregnant women. Viral loads should be monitored in HIV-infected pregnant women at the initial visit, 2 to 4 weeks after initiating or changing antiretroviral therapy, monthly until undetectable, and then at least every 3 months.[1] The recommended monitoring of viral load in pregnancy is more frequent than in nonpregnant women because of the need to lower viral load as rapidly as possible to decrease transmission risk. Viral load should also be assessed at approximately 34 to 36 weeks' gestation to inform decisions on the mode of delivery.[1] ARV-resistance testing should be performed on women who have persistently detectable plasma HIV RNA levels despite receiving cART. Because NRTIs may be associated with development of lactic acidosis, pregnant women receiving NRTIs should have hepatic enzymes and electrolytes monitored more frequently, and any new symptoms of potential hepatotoxicity should be evaluated thoroughly.[1]

Because of the physiologic changes during pregnancy such as hemodilution, the absolute CD4 count may decrease, thus the CD4 percentage tends to be more stable. Monitoring for complications of ARVs during pregnancy should be based on what is known about side effects of the drugs the woman is receiving (see Table 7 of the Perinatal Guidelines at http://www.aidsinfo.nih.gov/contentfiles/lvguidelines/perinatalgl.pdf, pp.62–76; accessed March 30, 2014).[1] Accurate dating of the pregnancy is important because scheduled cesarean deliveries for prevention of HIV transmission should be performed at 38 weeks' gestation before the onset of labor in the setting of maternal HIV viremia. Therefore, an ultrasonogram should be ordered as soon as possible to confirm the accuracy of the gestational age dating according to the last menstrual period.[1]

HIV-infected women receiving cART during pregnancy should receive a glucose screening with a standard, 1-hour, 50-g glucose loading test at 24 to 28 weeks of gestation. Some experts would perform earlier glucose screening in women with ongoing PI-based therapy initiated before pregnancy, similar to recommendations for women with a high-risk factor for glucose intolerance such as maternal obesity, advanced maternal age, and family history of diabetes mellitus.[1]

INTRAPARTUM CARE

AZT has been the mainstay of prevention of perinatal transmission since the PACTG 076 study was published in 1994, which included a regimen of intravenous AZT 2 mg/kg over 1 hour, followed by continuous infusion of 1 mg/kg/h until delivery for all HIV-infected women. This regimen, along with antepartum oral AZT and postexposure prophylaxis of oral AZT for the infant, was effective in reducing perinatal transmission by 67.5%.[38] The recommendation for use of intravenous AZT during delivery was made before cART regimens, which are now recommended for all HIV-infected pregnant women. Women who are receiving antepartum cART should continue this regimen on schedule during labor and before scheduled cesarean delivery. Intravenous AZT administration is recommended as part of cART for pregnant women with HIV RNA of at least 400 to 1000 copies/mL or unknown HIV RNA near delivery, regardless of antepartum regimen or mode of delivery.[1] Many experts choose to continue to give intravenous AZT to all HIV-positive women during labor and newborns regardless of the antepartum cART regimen, even though intrapartum prophylaxis was not associated with a lower risk of transmission among 2845 women with HIV RNA less than 400 copies/mL at delivery: 0.6% transmission with intrapartum prophylaxis versus 0% without intrapartum prophylaxis.[39] The 6-week neonatal component of the AZT chemoprophylaxis regimen is recommended for all HIV-exposed neonates to reduce perinatal transmission of HIV, preferably started within 6 to 12 hours of birth. Women receiving fixed-dose combination regimens that include AZT should have AZT administered intravenously during labor while other ARV components are continued orally. Obstetric procedures that increase maternal to fetal blood exchange should be avoided unless there are clear obstetric indications because of the increased risk of perinatal transmission, including: (1) artificial rupture of membranes, (2) use of fetal scalp electrode, and (3) assisted delivery with forceps of vacuum extractor, and/or episiotomy.[1]

For women who have received antepartum ARVs but have suboptimal viral suppression near delivery (ie, HIV RNA >1000 copies/mL), scheduled cesarean delivery is recommended to minimize perinatal transmission of HIV. Although perinatal HIV transmission can occur when the HIV RNA is less than 1000 copies/mL, there is no additional benefit to scheduled cesarean delivery when the HIV RNA is lower than 1000 copies/mL and therefore is not recommended. In the non-HIV infected woman, ACOG recommends that scheduled cesarean delivery should not occur until 39 weeks' gestation because of the neonatal morbidity associated with prematurity. However, to decrease the likelihood of rupture of membranes or labor, ACOG recommends scheduling cesarean delivery in HIV-infected women with HIV RNA >1000 copies/mL at 38 weeks to prevent prenatal HIV transmission. If the HIV RNA level is less than 1000 copies/mL and a cesarean delivery is indicated, cesarean delivery should be scheduled at 39 weeks' gestation.[1] Women with HIV RNA greater than 400 to 1000 copies/mL should have at least 3 hours of intravenous AZT before scheduled cesarean section or initiation of labor induction, because systemic and intracellular AZT levels reach a stable concentration after 3 hours of infusion (**Table 3**).[40]

Women of Unknown Human Immunodeficiency Virus Status Who Present in Labor

Women of unknown HIV status who present in labor should have rapid HIV-antibody testing performed and intravenous AZT initiated if the test is positive (without waiting for results of the confirmatory test), and infant AZT initiated. A confirmatory test should be done postpartum; if positive, 6 weeks of infant AZT is recommended, and if negative, the infant AZT can be stopped. In the postpartum period, along with confirmatory HIV antibody testing, these women should receive appropriate assessments as soon as possible to determine their health status, including CD4 cell count and HIV RNA viral load. Arrangements also should be made for establishing HIV care and providing ongoing psychosocial support after discharge. For HIV-infected women in labor who have not received antepartum ARVs, intravenous AZT during labor and 6 weeks of infant AZT is recommended. Some experts would combine the intravenous AZT intrapartum/6-week newborn AZT regimen with single-dose intrapartum/newborn nevirapine (NVP). Caution should be used when considering single-dose NVP in

Table 3
Use of antiretroviral drugs in pregnant HIV-1 infected women for maternal health and interventions to reduce perinatal HIV transmission

Clinical Situation	cART	IV AZT	Mode of Delivery	Timing of Delivery
VL <1000[a], no obstetric indication for cesarean delivery	Continue oral cART during labor and delivery	Not required	Vaginal delivery	Spontaneous or per obstetric indication
VL <1000, obstetric indication of cesarean delivery	Continue oral cART during delivery	Not required	Cesarean section	39 wk gestation per routine obstetric care
VL >1000	Continue cART without oral AZT during delivery	Required	Cesarean section	38 wk (before the onset of labor)
VL unknown	Continue cART without oral AZT if previously started	Required	Cesarean section	38 wk (before the onset of labor)

Abbreviation: cART, combination antiretroviral therapy.
[a] VL<1000 = HIV-RNA viral load level less than 1000 copies/mL.

women with high CD4 counts because of the theoretical risk of hepatotoxicity. If single-dose NVP is given (alone or in combination with AZT), consideration should be given to adding 3TC during labor and maternal AZT/3TC for 7 days postpartum or longer, which may reduce development of NVP resistance in the woman.[1] If the mother is found to have HIV RNA greater than 1000 copies/mL around delivery, some experts now recommend treatment doses of ART for the infant. However, optimal treatment of the newborn in the first 6 weeks of life remains controversial, and expert consultation is recommended.

Special Intrapartum Considerations

Women experiencing postpartum hemorrhage resulting from uterine atony are often managed with oral or intramuscular methergine as a first-line agent. However, methergine should not be coadministered with drugs that are potent CYP3A4 enzyme inhibitors, including PIs. The concomitant use of ergotamines and these CYP3A4-inhibiting drugs has been associated with exaggerated vasoconstrictive responses. If alternative treatments for postpartum hemorrhages are not available, methergine should be used in a low a dose and for as short a time as possible. By contrast, additional doses of methergine or other uterotonic agents may be needed when drugs that are CYP3A4 inducers, such as NVP, efavirenz, and etravirine, are used because of the potential for decreased methergine levels and an inadequate treatment effect.[1]

POSTPARTUM CARE

The postpartum period provides an excellent opportunity to optimize women's health care, particularly in HIV-infected women who often face multiple health-related and psychosocial challenges. Postpartum care for all HIV-infected women includes HIV, gynecologic, and obstetric care, in addition to family planning and mental health services. Some women require substance abuse treatment and support services. Women who receive family planning counseling during prenatal care are more likely to use effective contraception postpartum.[41] In countries where alternatives to breast-feeding are safe and affordable, breastfeeding is not recommended for HIV-infected women, regardless of their cART status. Because non-breastfeeding women ovulate more rapidly than women who are exclusively breastfeeding, contraception and family planning services are important immediately post-partum.[1] **Table 1** summarizes specific issues regarding the use of contraceptives in HIV-infected women.

All women who were started on cART during pregnancy should be counseled and encouraged to continue these ARVs after delivery given the current recommendations for ART, especially if their nadir CD4 counts are less than 500 cells/mm[3]. HIV viral load rebound has been noted with ART changes and discontinuations in the postpartum period.[42] The risks and benefits of stopping combination ART in women with high CD4 counts is currently under investigation. To avoid ARV resistance, women using an NNRTI-based regimen and who plan to stop ARV prophylaxis after delivery should consider continuing the other ARVs for at least 7 days while stopping the NNRTI.[1]

Infant Antiretroviral Prophylaxis

All HIV-exposed infants should receive postpartum postexposure prophylaxis of 6 weeks of oral AZT to reduce perinatal transmission. The dosing of the oral AZT is based on the gestational age and weight of the infant at birth. The risk of transmission is higher with increased maternal viral load at delivery, lack of antepartum or intrapartum ARV prophylaxis, infection of the mother with a known ARV-resistant virus, mode of delivery, and gestational age at delivery. Most experts believe that in situations with increased risks, infant ARV prophylaxis should include additional ARVs. **Table 4** shows infant prophylaxis recommendations in specific clinical scenarios; however, there is a paucity of data on these clinical situations, and each situation needs to be considered individually and in consultation with a pediatric HIV specialist.[1]

The National Perinatal HIV Hotline (1-888-448-8765) provides free clinical consultation to providers caring for HIV-infected pregnant women and their infants, and should be liberally used especially in clinical situations where strong recommendations are limited.

Table 4
Clinical scenarios and recommendations regarding ARV prophylaxis for infants

Clinical Scenario	Recommendations
Women who have not received antepartum or only intrapartum ARV prophylaxis	6 wk oral AZT, plus 3 doses of nevirapine at birth, 48 h and 96 h. Some experts may recommend treatment doses of antiretroviral therapy. As optimal treatment of the newborn in the first 6 wk of life is controversial, consultation with a pediatric HIV specialist is recommended
Women who have received antepartum ARV prophylaxis but have suboptimal viral suppression	6 wk oral AZT with consideration of combination infant prophylaxis regimen after consulting with pediatric HIV specialist
Women with ARV-resistant virus	The optimal prophylactic regimen is unknown and consultation with a pediatric HIV specialist is recommended. 6 wk oral AZT with consideration for combination ARV drugs selected based on maternal ARV-resistance patterns

Data from Panel on Treatment of HIV-Infected Pregnant Women and Prevention of Perinatal Transmission. Recommendations for use of antiretroviral drugs in pregnant HIV-1-infected women for maternal health and interventions to reduce perinatal HIV transmission in the United States. Department of Health and Human Services. Available at: http://aidsinfo.nih.gov/contentfiles/lvguidelines/perinatalgl.pdf. Accessed March 14, 2014.

REFERENCES

1. Panel on Treatment of HIV-Infected Pregnant Women and Prevention of Perinatal Transmission. Recommendations for use of antiretroviral drugs in pregnant HIV-1-infected women for maternal health and interventions to reduce perinatal HIV transmission in the United States. Department of Health and Human Services. Available at: http://aidsinfo.nih.gov/contentfiles/lvguidelines/PerinatalGL.pdf. Accessed March 30, 2014.
2. Johnson K, Posner SF, Biermann J, et al. Recommendations to improve preconception health and health care–United States. A report of the CDC/ATSDR Preconception Care Work Group and the Select Panel on Preconception Care. MMWR Recomm Rep 2006;55(RR-6):1–23.
3. American Congress of Obstetricians and Gynecologists (ACOG). Gynecological care for women with human immunodeficiency virus. Practice bulletin. 2010. Available at: http://www.acog.org/%7E/media/Practice%20Bulletins/Committee%20on%20Practice%20Bulletins%20%13%20Gynecology/Public/pb117.pdf?dmc=1&ts=20121127T0544419938. Accessed March 30, 2014.
4. American Congress of Obstetricians and Gynecologists (ACOG). ACOG Committee Opinion number 313, September 2005. The importance of preconception care in the continuum of women's health care. Obstet Gynecol 2005; 106(3):665–6.
5. Squires KE, Hodder SL, Feinberg J, et al. Health needs of HIV-infected women in the United States: insights from the women living positive survey. AIDS Patient Care STDs 2011;25(5):279–85.
6. Finocchario-Kessler S, Dariotis JK, Sweat MD, et al. Do HIV-infected women want to discuss reproductive plans with providers, and are those conversations occurring? AIDS Patient Care STDs 2010;24(5):317–23.
7. Panozzo L, Battegay M, Friedl A, et al. High risk behaviour and fertility desires among heterosexual HIV-positive patients with a serodiscordant partner–two challenging issues. Swiss Med Wkly 2003;133(7–8):124–7.
8. Sharma A, Feldman JG, Golub ET, et al. Live birth patterns among human immunodeficiency virus-infected women before and after the availability of highly active antiretroviral therapy. Am J Obstet Gynecol 2007;196(6):541.e1–6.
9. Finer LB, Zolna MR. Unintended pregnancy in the United States: incidence and disparities, 2006. Contraception 2011;84(5):478–85.
10. Massad LS, Springer G, Jacobson L, et al. Pregnancy rates and predictors of conception, miscarriage and abortion in US women with HIV. AIDS 2004;18(2):281–6.
11. Craft SM, Delaney RO, Bautista DT, et al. Pregnancy decisions among women with HIV. AIDS Behav 2007;11(6):927–35.
12. Cohn SE, Umbleja T, Mrus J, et al. Prior illicit drug use and missed prenatal vitamins predict nonadherence to antiretroviral therapy in pregnancy: adherence analysis A5084. AIDS Patient Care STDs 2008;22(1):29–40.
13. Hoyt MJ, Storm DS, Aaron E, et al. Preconception and contraceptive care for women living with HIV. Infect Dis Obstet Gynecol 2012;2012:604183.
14. Grady WR, Klepinger DH, Nelson-Wally A. Contraceptive characteristics: the perceptions and priorities of men and women. Fam Plann Perspect 1999;31(4):168–75.
15. Edwards JE, Oldman A, Smith L, et al. Women's knowledge of, and attitudes to, contraceptive effectiveness and adverse health effects. Br J Fam Plann 2000; 26(2):73–80.

16. Sadana R, Snow R. Balancing effectiveness, side-effects and work: women's perceptions and experiences with modern contraceptive technology in Cambodia. Soc Sci Med 1999;49(3):343–58.

17. World Health Organization/Department of Reproductive Health and Research (WHO/RHR), Johns Hopkins Bloomberg School of Public Health (JHSPH)/Center for Communication Programs (CCP). Family planning: a global handbook for providers. Baltimore (MD), Geneva (Switzerland): CCP and WHO; 2007.

18. Centers for Disease Control and Prevention. Effectiveness of family planning methods. Available at: http://www.cdc.gov/reproductivehealth/UnintendedPregnancy/PDF/Contraceptive_methods_508.pdf. Accessed March 30, 2014.

19. Centers for Disease Control and Prevention (CDC). US medical eligibility criteria for contraceptive use, 2010. MMWR Morb Mortal Wkly Rep 2010;59(4):1–86.

20. Coleman JS, Mwachari C, Balkus J, et al. Effect of the levonorgestrel intrauterine device on genital HIV-1 RNA shedding among HIV-1-infected women not taking antiretroviral therapy in Nairobi, Kenya. J Acquir Immune Defic Syndr 2013;63(2):245–8.

21. Phillips SJ, Curtis KM, Polis CB. Effect of hormonal contraceptive methods on HIV disease progression: a systematic review. AIDS 2013;27(5):787–94.

22. Stringer EM, Giganti M, Carter RJ, et al. Hormonal contraception and HIV disease progression: a multicountry cohort analysis of the MTCT-Plus Initiative. AIDS 2009;23(Suppl 1):S69–77.

23. Polis CB, Curtis KM. Use of hormonal contraceptives and HIV acquisition in women: a systematic review of the epidemiological evidence. Lancet Infect Dis 2013;13(9):797–808.

24. Baeten JM, Benki S, Chohan V, et al. Hormonal contraceptive use, herpes simplex virus infection, and risk of HIV-1 acquisition among Kenyan women. AIDS 2007;21(13):1771–7.

25. Morrison CS, Chen PL, Kwok C, et al. Hormonal contraception and HIV acquisition: reanalysis using marginal structural modeling. AIDS 2010;24(11):1778–81.

26. Heffron R, Donnell D, Rees H, et al. Use of hormonal contraceptives and risk of HIV-1 transmission: a prospective cohort study. Lancet Infect Dis 2012;12(1):19–26.

27. World Health Organization. Hormonal contraception and HIV: technical statement. 2012. Available at: http://whqlibdoc.who.int/hq/2012/WHO_RHR_12.08_eng.pdf?ua=1. Accessed March 30, 2014.

28. Tseng A, Hills-Nieminen C. Drug interactions between antiretrovirals and hormonal contraceptives. Expert Opin Drug Metab Toxicol 2013;9(5):559–72.

29. Robinson JA, Jamshidi R, Burke AE. Contraception for the HIV-positive woman: a review of interactions between hormonal contraception and antiretroviral therapy. Infect Dis Obstet Gynecol 2012;2012:890160.

30. Cohn SE, Park JG, Watts DH, et al. Depo-medroxyprogesterone in women on antiretroviral therapy: effective contraception and lack of clinically significant interactions. Clin Pharmacol Ther 2007;81(2):222–7.

31. Nattabi B, Li J, Thompson SC, et al. A systematic review of factors influencing fertility desires and intentions among people living with HIV/AIDS: implications for policy and service delivery. AIDS Behav 2009;13(5):949–68.

32. Lockman S, Hughes MD, McIntyre J, et al. Antiretroviral therapies in women after single-dose nevirapine exposure. N Engl J Med 2010;363(16):1499–509.

33. Townsend CL, Cortina-Borja M, Peckham CS, et al. Low rates of mother-to-child transmission of HIV following effective pregnancy interventions in the United Kingdom and Ireland, 2000-2006. AIDS 2008;22(8):973–81.

34. Tubiana R, Le Chenadec J, Rouzioux C, et al. Factors associated with mother-to-child transmission of HIV-1 despite a maternal viral load <500 copies/ml at delivery: a case-control study nested in the French perinatal cohort (EPF-ANRS CO1). Clin Infect Dis 2010;50(4):585–96.

35. Panel on Antiretroviral Guidelines for Adults and Adolescents. Guidelines for the use of antiretroviral agents in HIV-1-infected adults and adolescents. Department of Health and Human Services. Available at: http://aidsinfo.nih.gov/contentfiles/lvguidelines/AdultandAdolescentGL.pdf. Tables 15a, 15b, and 15d. Accessed March 29, 2014.

36. Grinsztejn B, Nguyen BY, Katlama C, et al. Safety and efficacy of the HIV-1 integrase inhibitor raltegravir (MK-0518) in treatment-experienced patients with multidrug-resistant virus: a phase II randomised controlled trial. Lancet 2007; 369(9569):1261–9.

37. Ford N, Calmy A, Mofenson L. Safety of efavirenz in the first trimester of pregnancy: an updated systematic review and meta-analysis. AIDS 2011;25(18): 2301–4.

38. Connor EM, Sperling RS, Gelber R, et al. Reduction of maternal-infant transmission of human immunodeficiency virus type 1 with zidovudine treatment. Pediatric AIDS Clinical Trials Group Protocol 076 Study immunodeficiency Group. N Engl J Med 1994;331(18):1173–80.

39. Warszawski J, Tubiana R, Le Chenadec J, et al. Mother-to-child HIV transmission despite antiretroviral therapy in the ANRS French Perinatal Cohort. AIDS 2008; 22(2):289–99.

40. Rodman JH, Flynn PM, Robbins B, et al. Systemic pharmacokinetics and cellular pharmacology of zidovudine in human virus type 1-infected women and newborn infants. J Infect Dis 1999;180(6):1844–50.

41. Jackson E. Controversies in postpartum contraception: when is it safe to start oral contraceptives after childbirth? Thromb Res 2011;127(Suppl 3):S35–9.

42. Sha BE, Tierney C, Cohn SE, et al. Postpartum viral load rebound in HIV-1-infected women treated with highly active antiretroviral therapy: AIDS Clinical Trials Group Protocol A5150. HIV Clin Trials 2011;12(1):9–23.

43. Tivicay (dolutegravir) [package insert]. Available at: http://www.accessdata.fda.gov/drugsatfda_docs/label/2013/204790lbl.pdf. Accessed March 15, 2014.

Rationale and Evidence for Human Immunodeficiency Virus Treatment as Prevention at the Individual and Population Levels

Christopher J. Hoffmann, MD, MPH[a], Joel E. Gallant, MD, MPH[a,b],*

KEYWORDS

- HIV • Antiretroviral therapy • Prevention • TasP • Treatment as prevention
- Adherence • HIV testing • Epidemic

KEY POINTS

- The risk of HIV transmission to a sexual partner is reduced 96% if the HIV-infected partner is on ART, and maybe close to 100% if the infected partner has achieved an undetectable viral load through the use of antiretroviral therapy.
- Initiation of HIV treatment with the safe and well-tolerated antiretroviral agents available in high-income countries is likely to benefit patients regardless of CD4 count.
- Scale-up of voluntary HIV screening followed by treatment of all HIV-infected individuals, along with other prevention methods, could have a significant public health impact, potentially slowing or stopping the HIV epidemic.
- Current levels of HIV testing and treatment are inadequate to achieve significant population-level prevention.

INTRODUCTION

Efforts to halt the human immunodeficiency virus (HIV) epidemic have failed on a population level. Despite attention and resources, the global HIV pandemic has been marked by an increasing number of people living with HIV.[1] Overall an estimated 35 million individuals were living with HIV globally in 2012, an increase of 5 million from 10 years earlier. Although the global HIV prevalence is 0.8%, in some countries the prevalence is much higher. For example, in Swaziland 26% of the adult population is HIV infected.[2]

[a] Division of Infectious Diseases, Department of Medicine, Johns Hopkins University School of Medicine, 725 North Wolfe Street, Room 226, Baltimore, MD 21205, USA; [b] Department of Specialty Services, Southwest CARE Center, 649 Harkle Road, Suite E, Sante Fe, NM 87505, USA
* Corresponding author. 649 Harkle Road, Suite E, Santa Fe, NM 87505.
E-mail address: jgallant@southwestcare.org

Infect Dis Clin N Am 28 (2014) 549–561
http://dx.doi.org/10.1016/j.idc.2014.08.003
0891-5520/14/$ – see front matter © 2014 Elsevier Inc. All rights reserved.

id.theclinics.com

In both high- and low-prevalence countries, HIV distribution varies considerably by population group. For example, sex workers, men who have sex with men (MSM), and injection drug users (IDU) are consistently affected out of proportion to the background population. In the United States, nearly one quarter of black MSM are infected, and the overall prevalence among black men in Washington, DC, is 7%.[3] In Africa, the HIV prevalence among MSM is often twice that of the non-MSM male population.[4–6] Additional vulnerable groups, such as impoverished young women, are also at high risk for HIV infection. Among young women living in informal settlements in South Africa, the annual HIV incidence is between 5% and 15%.[4,7]

High HIV incidence has persisted despite substantial prevention efforts. The current situation reflects a failure to apply proven effective prevention approaches. The 3 notable exceptions have been the use of antiretrovirals for the prevention of mother-to-child transmission (PMTCT), condom promotion to reduce HIV infection among sex workers and their clients in Thailand,[8] and needle exchange to reduce incidence among IDU in inner-city settings.[9]

PMTCT has parallels with treatment as prevention (TasP). PMTCT uses antiretrovirals during pregnancy and post partum to reduce the risk of MTCT. On a population level, implementation of PMTCT programs has reduced transmission from about 35% to 1% to 5%.[10–12] The success of population-level implementation of PMTCT is a result of the intersection of global health funding that has made provision of services financially feasible and the time-limited intervention of PMTCT integrated within the medical management of pregnancy.

TasP has appeal with its parallels to PMTCT and its applicability to all types of epidemics, because it is presumed to interrupt heterosexual, MSM, IDU, and mother-to-child transmission. Evidence of the potential of ART to prevent HIV transmission has been present for at least a decade.[13] More recently, clinical trial evidence, increased ART availability, and the development of better tolerated ART agents have coalesced to the point that TasP is a now considered to be a realistic approach to reversing the HIV epidemic. This article reviews the data supporting the use of TasP on an individual level and on a population level.

THEORETIC BASIS: VIRAL LOAD AND HUMAN IMMUNODEFICIENCY VIRUS TRANSMISSION OBSERVATIONAL STUDIES

Untreated Individuals

The concentration of HIV in the blood correlates with the risk of both MTCT and sexual transmission.[14] An early study of 415 HIV-discordant couples in Uganda, in which the seropositive partner was not receiving ART, found no transmissions when the infected partner had a plasma viral load of less than 1500 copies/mL.[15] The rate of transmission increased progressively up to 23 per 100 person-years among partners of infected individuals with viral loads of greater than 50,000 copies/mL. A meta-analysis combining data from 10 serodiscordant partner studies reported a linear increase in transmission risk from 0.16 per 100 person-years for couples in which the infected partner had a viral load below 400 copies/mL to 9 per 100 person-years when the infected partner had a viral load of more than 50,000 copies/mL.[16] These transmission risk studies were based on "stable" discordant relationships and may underestimate transmission risks during sex with new or casual partners.[17]

Treated Individuals

Several studies have prospectively followed heterosexual couples in which 1 member of the couple was HIV infected and received ART and the other was seronegative. Among

5 studies providing a combined 1000 person-years of follow-up and 5 incident infections, the calculated transmission rate with the use of ART was 0.5 per 100 person-years.[16] This represents a markedly lower incidence than the 9 per 100 person-years that has been observed with partnerships in which the infected partner had a viral load of more than 50,000 copies/mL, but it still represents an important transmission risk.

What is unclear from these studies is whether the infected partner had a detectable viral load at the time of transmission; viral load data were not available in most of these studies. In addition, none of these studies confirmed that transmission occurred from within the partnership, because phylogenetic testing was not conducted. Thus, the estimate of 0.5 per 100 person-years may overestimate the risk for a stable, discordant couple if the infected partner is adherent to a suppressive ART regimen. Preliminary results from a European study of heterosexual and MSM couples suggest a very low risk of transmission when the HIV-infected partner is on ART with a viral load of <200 c/mL; no linked transmission events have been identified as of 2014.[18] This study includes a substantial number of couples engaging in condomless sex (767); 30% of these couples are MSM within which 40% of the HIV-negative partners engaged in condomless receptive anal sex with ejaculation, which is associated with a higher risk of transmission than vaginal sex or insertive anal sex. The 95% confidence bound around the risk of transmission during receptive anal sex ranged from zero to 0.96 transmissions per 100 couple-years. If no transmission events are identified through the duration of the study (to be completed in 2017), the wide confidence interval will become narrower.

Plasma Versus Genital Fluid Human Immunodeficiency Virus Concentration and Transmission

One of the concerns regarding the transmission safety of unprotected sex despite an undetectable plasma viral load is the discrepancy between plasma and genital fluid HIV levels. In untreated infection, both plasma and genital HIV concentrations peak during acute infection, with genital levels remaining elevated for several months longer than plasma levels.[19,20] Following the acute phase, genital fluid concentrations vary considerably more than plasma levels.[19] Among individuals treated with ART and achieving an undetectable plasma viral load, genital HIV concentration tends to follow the plasma level, but the correlation is imperfect. Among men on ART with undetectable plasma HIV levels, semen levels of up to 16,000 copies/mL have been observed.[21]

A single study has compared transmission risk by genital and plasma viral load among untreated individuals in discordant couples.[22] The investigators found a stronger correlation with transmission and genital viral load than plasma viral load.

CLINICAL TRIALS

The HIV Prevention Trials Network (HPTN) 052 study was a rigorous evaluation of the hypothesis that the use of ART by an HIV-infected individual could prevent transmission to an uninfected partner.[23] HPTN 052 enrolled discordant couples (partners for at least 3 months) in 9 countries. The infected partners had to have a CD4 count between 350 and 550 cells/mm^3 and were randomized to initiate ART either at study entry or after the CD4 count fell to below 250 cells/mm^3, consistent with local guidelines at the time. Seronegative partners underwent quarterly testing, and if found to be positive their viral strain was compared phylogenetically with their partner's strain. At each study visit, risk reduction and condom use messages were provided.

A total of 1763 couples (98% heterosexual) were enrolled and followed for a total of 3152 person-years until the study was unblinded and all infected participants were offered ART (based on a prespecified data monitoring and safety board stop decision rule). During follow-up before study unblinding, 39 transmission events occurred. Four events (incidence of 0.3 per 100 person-years) occurred in the early therapy group and 35 (incidence of 2.2 per 100 person-years) in the delayed therapy group. Of the 4 events in the early therapy group, only one was phylogenetically linked to the partner; the other 3 were unlinked and presumably came from outside the partnership. This represented a 96% protection from transmission. The 1 linked transmission occurred within 3 months of initiation of ART, presumably before virologic control had been achieved.

These results, with robust viral load data and incident infection monitoring from a randomized population, provide definitive evidence that use of ART substantially decreases HIV transmission. Importantly, these results reflect a heterosexual population. Receptive anal sex carries a higher risk for HIV acquisition than receptive or insertive vaginal sex, insertive anal sex, or oral sex and may not be as effectively eliminated by suppression of plasma viral load. However, the preliminary results from the PARTNER observational study, described above, suggest that ART may be nearly as protective or equally protective among MSM couples.

INDIVIDUAL DECISION MAKING

In 2008, 4 prominent Swiss HIV physicians issued what has been referred to as "the Swiss Statement," which suggested that condom use was unnecessary within discordant couples if the infected partners had undetectable HIV viral loads for more than 6 months.[24] This position was based on 2 assumptions: (1) The risk of transmission was felt to be less than 1 in 100,000, which was considered to be an acceptable risk and (2) the use of viral suppression as a means to minimize transmission would increase adherence to ART.

No published guidelines have taken a similarly strong stance on this issue. The closest is the British HIV Association guidelines for postexposure prophylaxis (PEP). These guidelines recommend PEP after an exposure to an individual with an undetectable viral load in only 1 situation: Receptive anal sex. In the British HIV Association guidelines, PEP is not recommended after HIV exposure through insertive anal sex or vaginal sex if the HIV-infected individual has an undetectable viral load.[25] Guidelines for sexual HIV prevention, including those from the US Centers for Disease Control and Prevention, continue to recommend condom use even within a discordant partnership in which the infected partner has an undetectable viral load, regardless of sexual practice (vaginal insertive, anal receptive, etc).[26]

POPULATION-LEVEL PREVENTION: MODELING OF TREATMENT AS PREVENTION

Observational studies and the HPTN 052 clinical trial have confirmed the power of ART to prevent HIV transmission on an individual level. Less is known about the impact of ART on a population level, but several mathematical modeling studies suggest that rapid scale up of ART could effectively eliminate transmission.

A mathematical model published in 2009 galvanized thinking about the potential of widespread ART to reverse the HIV epidemic.[27] The authors modeled the effect of universal ART on the South African epidemic. They assumed annual testing for all HIV-undiagnosed individuals followed by immediate ART initiation. After ART initiation, the authors assumed that approximately 3% of patients would leave care in the first year followed by 1.5% in all subsequent years. All transmission was assumed to be heterosexual, and sexual mixing was assumed to be evenly distributed throughout the population. Based on these assumptions and assuming immediate scale up, the authors calculated that over a period of 10 years the epidemic could be eliminated, defined as an incidence below 1 infection per 1000 person-years (**Fig. 1**).

Additional models have also suggested that HIV incidence can be brought to less than 1 infection per 1000 person-years with annual HIV testing and immediate ART, assuming coverage of 90% of HIV-infected individuals. A study comparing models concluded that even with more realistic assumptions regarding loss from care and virologic failure than used in the 2009 model, elimination is possible over 20 to 30 years.[28]

POPULATION-BASED PREVENTION ECOLOGICAL STUDIES

An ecological study from San Francisco reflecting a largely MSM epidemic identified a reduction in new infections from 798 in 2004 to 434 in 2008.[29] This correlated with increased ART coverage and a decrease in the median viral load of all HIV-diagnosed individuals in San Francisco. The measure of median viral load among diagnosed individuals is referred to as the "community viral load" and is an indication of the proportion of individuals receiving suppressive ART among all individuals with known HIV infection. Another ecological study, also set in San Francisco and also reflecting a mostly MSM epidemic, estimated a 60% decline in infectivity comparing the period before widespread ART use (1994–1995) with a period in which ART use was widespread (1997–1999).[30]

In a mostly IDU epidemic in Vancouver, Canada, the number of newly diagnosed individuals declined between 1996 and 2012 during a period of expansion in ART coverage. During this period, the number of individuals with known HIV receiving ART increased from 11% to 57%.[31] The researchers estimated a 42% reduction in HIV incidence, correlating with the increase in ART coverage. The San Francisco and Vancouver studies followed a gradual change in ART coverage that may have coincided with other important changes that could also have led to a decline in HIV incidence.

A study from a research site in South Africa compared HIV incidence by the proportion of the community receiving ART by location and time from 2005 to 2011. The

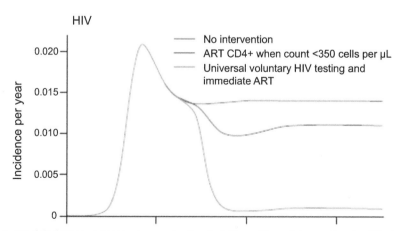

Fig. 1. Modeled HIV incidence per year for South Africa with no intervention (*red line*), ART initiation in all individuals with a CD4 count of less than 350 cells/mm³ (*blue line*), and universal HIV testing and immediate ART (*green line*). (*From* Granich RM, Gilks CF, Dye C, et al. Universal voluntary HIV testing with immediate antiretroviral therapy as a strategy for elimination of HIV transmission: a mathematical model. Lancet 2009;373:51; with permission.)

investigators had access to individual HIV test results, behavioral data, and ART coverage. Using these data, the investigators calculated an adjusted hazard ratio of HIV infection by the proportion of infected people receiving ART living in a 3-km radius of each uninfected adult in the population.[32] The authors reported a 38% reduction in HIV incidence among individuals in an area with 30% to 40% ART coverage compared with areas with less than 10% coverage (**Fig. 2**).

These ecological studies provide important preliminary evidence that TasP may have a substantial population-level impact. Several large studies are underway in southern Africa to test the concept of TasP to eliminate HIV transmission.[33,34]

BALANCING THE INDIVIDUAL WITH THE POPULATION

For ART to have meaningful population-level impact, at least 80% to 90% of infected individuals must be receiving ART. This raises important questions regarding risk–benefit considerations to individuals, especially those with higher CD4 counts. There is strong evidence that ART is beneficial when initiated at CD4 counts less than 350 cells/mm^3.[35] The SMART study compared initiation of ART at a CD4 count of 350 cells/mm^3 with ART initiation at 350 cells/mm^3 with interruption when the CD4 count rose above 350 cells/mm^3 and re-initiation when the CD4 count dropped below 250 cells/mm^3. The investigators hypothesized that these structured treatment interruptions would reduce what were assumed to be ART-associated complications, such as liver, kidney, and heart disease, while avoiding HIV-associated illnesses. In fact, they found an increase in all illnesses, including liver, kidney, and heart complications, as well as opportunistic illnesses, among participants in the structured treatment interruption arm. This study cemented the idea that ART prevents illnesses beyond those associated with low CD4 counts.

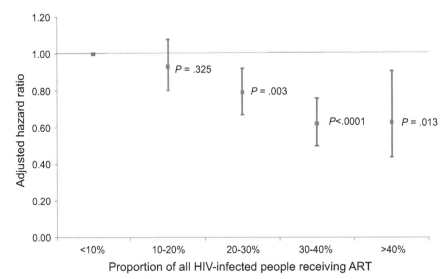

Fig. 2. Multivariable analysis showing HIV-uninfected individual's adjusted hazard ratio of HIV infection, with 95% CI bands, by community proportion of HIV-infected individuals receiving ART. (*From* Tanser F, Barnighausen T, Grapsa E, et al. High coverage of ART associated with decline in risk of HIV acquisition in rural KwaZulu-Natal, South Africa. Science 2013;339:968; with permission.)

After the SMART study, a smaller study in Haiti randomized 816 HIV-infected participants with CD4 counts between 200 and 350 cells/mm³ to either initiate ART immediately or to wait until the CD4 count dropped below 200 cells/mm³.[36] During approximately 21 months of observation, there were 23 deaths in the standard treatment group and 6 in the early treatment group (hazard ratio, 4.0), and a significantly greater incidence of tuberculosis in the standard treatment group. This study reinforced the health benefit of initiating ART at least using a 350 cells/mm³ threshold, and influenced World Health Organization guidelines for use of ART in low- and middle-income countries.

Large observational studies have explored the health benefit of ART initiation at higher CD4 counts. In 1 study that included records from 17,000 patients from clinics in North America, the investigators compared ART initiation at CD4 counts between 351 and 500 cells/mm³ with starting at a CD4 count below 350 cells/mm³.[37] There was a 69% increase in the risk of death in the deferred group. A second analysis compared starting ART with CD4 counts greater than 500 cells/mm³ with starting ART below that threshold and estimated a 94% increase in risk of death with delayed initiation.

Another large study with clinical and research data on 21,000 patients from cohorts in Europe and North America compared patient outcomes among patients by CD4 count at ART initiation.[38] In that study, there was improved survival with initiation at a CD4 count of more than 351 cells/mm³, but no added survival benefit when starting at a CD4 count between 451 and 550 cells/mm³ versus 351 and 450 cells/mm³. Delaying until the CD4 count was between 251 and 350 cells/mm³ increased mortality and AIDS events by 28%.

These studies provide strong evidence for a health benefit of initiating ART at a threshold of 350 cells/mm³ and possibly up to 450 or 500 cells/mm³. However, the question of whether there is a clinical benefit to starting ART at higher CD4 counts remains unanswered and is being investigated in an ongoing clinical trial (START study; available from http://www.clinicaltrials.gov; NCT00867048).

An additional consideration regarding benefits of very early ART is the potential for improving immune control of HIV and reducing immune cell loss. Several studies have evaluated the use of ART in acute or early HIV infection (within 6 months of infection) to improve long-term CD4 count and reduce the untreated viral load; these studies have had mixed results.[39] Other studies have evaluated the effect of early ART on specific immune cell subsets and suggested subset preservation.[40] The health benefits from initiating ART during acute HIV infection remain unknown.

If ART is deferred until the CD4 count has fallen to a threshold of 350 or 500 cells/mm³, the total time a patient spends before initiating ART may be relatively short when measured from time of HIV acquisition. Several studies of acute or early HIV have quantified the time from acute infection to a CD4 count of less than 500 cells/mm³. One study reported a median time of 1.2 years.[41] This suggests that within 1 or 2 years after HIV infection, most individuals will have reached a CD4 count of less than 500 cells/mm³. Thus, over the lifetime of a patient, earlier ART initiation would result in only a marginal increase in total time on ART.

However, in a subset of HIV-infected individuals CD4 count declines slowly, suggesting that in this population early initiation of ART might not be as beneficial. This is most pronounced among long-term nonprogressors—individuals who maintain a CD4 count above 500 cells/mm³ for more than 8 to 10 years without ART. Approximately 5% of individuals with HIV are long-term nonprogressors.[42,43] At present, it is unclear whether ART initiation at CD4 counts above 500 cells/mm³ benefits long-term nonprogressors. These patients cannot be identified prospectively as they are defined as fitting into the category only after longitudinal follow-up.

The US Department of Health and Human Services (DHHS) and International Antiviral Society-USA (IAS-USA) guidelines now recommend initiation of ART in all patients regardless of CD4 count, based on a combination of the results of the large treatment cohorts, the prevention data from HPTN 052, the safety and tolerability of contemporary ART regimens, and evidence that ART reduces inflammation and immune activation that may contribute to long-term morbidity and mortality.[44,45] The European AIDS Clinical Society (EACS) October 2013 guidelines, British HIV Association (BHIVA), and World Health Organization 2013 adult ART guidelines all recommend ART initiation with a CD4 count either at 350 or 500 cells/mm^3.[46–48] The variation in guidelines partially reflects the limited data on ART benefits at higher CD4 counts, the potential adverse events, and the relative weight guideline committees presumably placed on both cost and the preventive benefits of ART.

Importantly, data that influenced the US recommendations for universal ART cannot be directly extrapolated to low- and middle-income countries where treatment resources are more limited. In many parts of the world, more toxic drugs such as stavudine, zidovudine, and didanosine are still being widely used for initial therapy, viral load testing is not widely available, drug stock outs are common, and options for second-line therapy and beyond are limited and are chosen empirically without access to resistance testing. In such settings, the public health benefit of early initiation of ART may be offset by the potential harm to individuals who are at low risk of HIV-associated morbidity and mortality.[49] For early ART to be ethical, it is important to address the disparities between the quality of care between resource-rich and resource-limited settings.

TREATMENT AS PREVENTION AND THE HUMAN IMMUNODEFICIENCY VIRUS PREVENTION LANDSCAPE

TasP is an essential component of a prevention strategy for ending the HIV epidemic. However, even with sufficient financial resources and adequate uptake of HIV testing and ART, it will be most effective in the context of additional prevention approaches. Integrated and rational use of multiple prevention approaches is referred to as "combination prevention."[50] By weaving together multiple approaches, combination prevention can address limitations of each approach and can target specific transmission dynamics within a population.

An important limitation of TasP is that it is aimed entirely at the HIV-infected partner. Additional approaches are needed to protect and empower HIV-uninfected individuals. This is critical in situations of casual sex in which an uninfected individual may not know his or her partner's HIV status, treatment status, or viral load. It is also critical in situations in which the uninfected partner is not empowered to insist or rely on HIV status disclosure or an undetectable viral load as a condition for sex.

Several methods are effective for HIV-uninfected individuals to reduce the risk of infection that do not depend on partner participation. These include pre-exposure prophylaxis, male medical circumcision, and potentially microbicides. PEP is also an important method for use by HIV-uninfected individuals, but its role is limited to specific situations including rape, condom failure, and other unexpected situations of exposure to body fluids from an individual with known or possible HIV infection. Additional important HIV prevention approaches include behavior change and condom use, needle exchange and opioid substitution, and PMTCT. Further discussion of specific prevention approaches is addressed elsewhere.

CHALLENGES

The first challenge to population-level TasP is ensuring that HIV infection is diagnosed early. An effective and sustained testing system is needed to identify individuals during, or as soon as possible after, acute HIV infection to minimize further cycles of transmission. The optimal frequency of testing depends on the sexual mixing and transmission dynamics of that population. For example, a subpopulation in which the majority of transmission is believed to occur during the early infection period, as described in Montreal among MSM,[51] must have effective means to identify acutely infected individuals. In other settings, acute HIV infection may play a minor role in maintaining the epidemic.[52] In a situation in which acute infection is less of a driver of the epidemic, high levels of coverage of at risk individuals with HIV testing, over time, is more critical than frequent testing of the most at-risk population.

At present, there is a failure of early HIV diagnosis in both higher and lower risk populations and in both high-income and low- and middle-income countries. Among MSM in London, an estimated 25% are unaware of their HIV status and in the United States one third of black MSM are unaware of being infected.[53,54] In southern Africa, an estimated 50% of adults have never been tested for HIV.[55,56]

Clearly, current levels of testing are not achieving early diagnosis in a substantial number of persons. To overcome the testing gap, concerted efforts are needed to increase voluntary HIV counseling and testing, especially among those at most risk for HIV, and to increase provider-initiated testing. The US Preventive Services Task Force (USPSTF) recommends that clinicians test for HIV among all adolescents and adults aged 15 to 65 years and all pregnant women. In addition, individuals younger than 15 and older than 65 who are at increased risk for HIV should be tested.[57] The USPSTF recommends testing at least once for lower risk individuals and testing every 1 to 5 years for individuals at higher risk for HIV infection. The US Centers for Disease Control and Prevention (CDC) have similar guidelines.[58]

Achieving effective linkage-to-care and retention-in-care after diagnosis remains another challenge. The failures along the diagnosis to suppression cascade have been the subject of multiple reports.[59,60] The care cascade has been highlighted as a major barrier to effective implementation of TasP in both high-income and low- and middle-income settings. Once in care, the effectiveness of TasP depends on ART adherence. Effective and sustained prevention using ART depends on achieving and maintaining an undetectable viral load, which is essential for preventing transmission and avoiding drug resistance, which can be transmitted. Approaches to improving adherence are beyond the scope of this review, but need to be ongoing and coordinated with all components of care.[61]

Another part of the solution to the entry-into-care gap is to provide an integrated and functioning care delivery system that ensures an uninterrupted supply of medications, accessible and acceptable clinical facilities, and sufficient clinical staffing and organization to minimize delays in obtaining care.[49] A functioning system will help to prevent the emergence and transmission of drug resistant virus, which could complicate TasP, especially in lower resourced settings where resistance testing is unaffordable.[62]

Finally, the social stigma associated with HIV infection and the groups at greatest risk, including MSM, IDU, and commercial sex workers, remains a major barrier to HIV testing and care. Political and social leaders can assist in providing messages to reduce stigma.

Political will to channel resources now to achieve future savings is critically important. The infrastructure needed to stop the epidemic through TasP as a component of combination prevention will not come cheaply. Rational advocacy is essential to usher in the needed testing, linkage, and treatment services.

SUMMARY

The individual health benefits of ART, including early ART, are becoming clearer, and in resource-rich countries, the short- and long-term side effects of current ART regimens are minimal. Thus, US guidelines now recommend ART for the benefit of the patient regardless of CD4 count or viral load.

Maintaining an undetectable viral load through adherence to an ART regimen comes close to eliminating the risk of HIV transmission, leading the US HIV treatment guidelines to recommend universal ART to reduce HIV transmission. Achieving population-level control of the epidemic through TasP may be feasible, but requires the expenditure of considerable resources devoted to HIV testing, linkage to care, ART accessibility, and retention in care. Ongoing population-based studies evaluating the use of TasP, along with other prevention interventions, will provide valuable insight into the complexity and true cost of achieving meaningful ART coverage.

REFERENCES

1. Joint United Nations Programme on HIV/AIDS. Global report: UNAIDS report on the global AIDS epidemic 2013. Geneva (Switzerland): United Nations; 2013.
2. Joint United Nations Programme on HIV/AIDS (UNAIDS). Getting to zero: HIV in eastern & southern Africa. Geneva (Switzerland): United Nations; 2013.
3. Magnus M, Kuo I, Phillips G, et al. Elevated HIV prevalence despite lower rates of sexual risk behaviors among black men in the District of Columbia who have sex with men. AIDS Patient Care STDS 2010;24:615–22.
4. Tanser F, de OT, Maheu-Giroux M, et al. Concentrated HIV subepidemics in generalized epidemic settings. Curr Opin HIV AIDS 2014;9:115–25.
5. Wolf RC, Cheng AS, Kapesa L, et al. Building the evidence base for urgent action: HIV epidemiology and innovative programming for men who have sex with men in sub-Saharan Africa. J Int AIDS Soc 2013;16(Suppl 3):18903.
6. Beyrer C, Baral SD, van Griensven F, et al. Global epidemiology of HIV infection in men who have sex with men. Lancet 2012;380:367–77.
7. Nel A, Mabude Z, Smit J, et al. HIV incidence remains high in KwaZulu-Natal, South Africa: evidence from three districts. PLoS One 2012;7:e35278.
8. Kilmarx PH, Supawitkul S, Wankrairoj M, et al. Explosive spread and effective control of human immunodeficiency virus in northernmost Thailand: the epidemic in Chiang Rai province, 1988-99. AIDS 2000;14:2731–40.
9. Vlahov D, Junge B. The role of needle exchange programs in HIV prevention. Public Health Rep 1998;113(Suppl 1):75–80.
10. Mnyani CN, McIntyre JA. Preventing mother-to-child transmission of HIV. BJOG 2009;116(Suppl 1):71–6.
11. Townsend CL, Cortina-Borja M, Peckham CS, et al. Low rates of mother-to-child transmission of HIV following effective pregnancy interventions in the United Kingdom and Ireland, 2000-2006. AIDS 2008;22:973–81.
12. Motswere-Chirwa C, Voetsch A, Lu L, et al. Follow-Up of Infants Diagnosed with HIV - Early Infant Diagnosis Program, Francistown, Botswana, 2005-2012. MMWR Morb Mortal Wkly Rep 2014;63:158–60.
13. Velasco-Hernandez JX, Gershengorn HB, Blower SM. Could widespread use of combination antiretroviral therapy eradicate HIV epidemics? Lancet Infect Dis 2002;2:487–93.

14. Mofenson LM, Lambert JS, Stiehm ER, et al. Risk factors for perinatal transmission of human immunodeficiency virus type 1 in women treated with zidovudine. Pediatric AIDS Clinical Trials Group Study 185 Team. N Engl J Med 1999;341: 385–93.
15. Quinn TC, Wawer MJ, Sewankambo N, et al. Viral load and heterosexual transmission of human immunodeficiency virus type 1. Rakai Project Study Group. N Engl J Med 2000;342:921–9.
16. Attia S, Egger M, Muller M, et al. Sexual transmission of HIV according to viral load and antiretroviral therapy: systematic review and meta-analysis. AIDS 2009;23:1397–404.
17. Powers KA, Poole C, Pettifor AE, et al. Rethinking the heterosexual infectivity of HIV-1: a systematic review and meta-analysis. Lancet Infect Dis 2008;8:553–63.
18. Rodger A, Cambiano V, Vernazza P, et al. HIV transmission risk through condomless sex if the HIV+ partner is on suppressive ART. Conference on Retroviruses and Opportunistic Infections; Abstract 153LB. Boston, Massachusetts, March 3–6: 2014.
19. Pilcher CD, Joaki G, Hoffman IF, et al. Amplified transmission of HIV-1: comparison of HIV-1 concentrations in semen and blood during acute and chronic infection. AIDS 2007;21:1723–30.
20. Morrison CS, Demers K, Kwok C, et al. Plasma and cervical viral loads among Ugandan and Zimbabwean women during acute and early HIV-1 infection. AIDS 2010;24:573–82.
21. Sheth PM, Kovacs C, Kemal KS, et al. Persistent HIV RNA shedding in semen despite effective antiretroviral therapy. AIDS 2009;23:2050–4.
22. Baeten JM, Kahle E, Lingappa JR, et al. Genital HIV-1 RNA predicts risk of heterosexual HIV-1 transmission. Sci Transl Med 2011;3:77ra29.
23. Cohen MS, Chen YQ, McCauley M, et al. Prevention of HIV-1 infection with early antiretroviral therapy. N Engl J Med 2011;365:493–505.
24. Vernazza PL, Hirschel B, Bernasconi E, et al. Les personnes seropositives ne souffrant d'aucune autre MST et suivant un traitement antiretroviral efficace ne transmettent pas le VIH par voie sexuelle. Bull Med Suisse 2008;89:165–9.
25. Benn P, Fisher M, Kulasegaram R. UK guideline for the use of post-exposure prophylaxis for HIV following sexual exposure (2011). Int J STD AIDS 2011; 22:695–708.
26. Centers for Disease Control and Prevention. Preventing new HIV infections. 2014. 2-20-2014. Available at: www.cdc.gov.
27. Granich RM, Gilks CF, Dye C, et al. Universal voluntary HIV testing with immediate antiretroviral therapy as a strategy for elimination of HIV transmission: a mathematical model. Lancet 2009;373:48–57.
28. Hontelez JA, Lurie MN, Barnighausen T, et al. Elimination of HIV in South Africa through expanded access to antiretroviral therapy: a model comparison study. PLoS Med 2013;10:e1001534.
29. Das M, Chu PL, Santos GM, et al. Decreases in community viral load are accompanied by reductions in new HIV infections in San Francisco. PLoS One 2010;5: e11068.
30. Porco TC, Martin JN, Page-Shafer KA, et al. Decline in HIV infectivity following the introduction of highly active antiretroviral therapy. AIDS 2004;18:81–8.
31. Montaner JS, Lima VD, Harrigan PR, et al. Expansion of HAART coverage is associated with sustained decreases in HIV/AIDS morbidity, mortality and HIV transmission: the "HIV treatment as prevention" experience in a Canadian setting. PLoS One 2014;9:e87872.

32. Tanser F, Barnighausen T, Grapsa E, et al. High coverage of ART associated with decline in risk of HIV acquisition in rural KwaZulu-Natal, South Africa. Science 2013;339:966–71.

33. Iwuji CC, Orne-Gliemann J, Tanser F, et al. Evaluation of the impact of immediate versus WHO recommendations-guided antiretroviral therapy initiation on HIV incidence: the ANRS 12249 TasP (Treatment as Prevention) trial in Hlabisa sub-district, KwaZulu-Natal, South Africa: study protocol for a cluster randomised controlled trial. Trial 2013;14:230.

34. Vermund SH, Fidler SJ, Ayles H, et al. Can combination prevention strategies reduce HIV transmission in generalized epidemic settings in Africa? The HPTN 071 (PopART) study plan in South Africa and Zambia. J Acquir Immune Defic Syndr 2013;63(Suppl 2):S221–7.

35. El-Sadr WM, Lundgren JD, Neaton JD, et al. CD4+ count-guided interruption of antiretroviral treatment. N Engl J Med 2006;355:2283–96.

36. Severe P, Juste MA, Ambroise A, et al. Early versus standard antiretroviral therapy for HIV-infected adults in Haiti. N Engl J Med 2010;363:257–65.

37. Kitahata MM, Gange SJ, Abraham AG, et al. Effect of early versus deferred antiretroviral therapy for HIV on survival. N Engl J Med 2009;360:1815–26.

38. Sterne JA, May M, Costagliola D, et al. Timing of initiation of antiretroviral therapy in AIDS-free HIV-1-infected patients: a collaborative analysis of 18 HIV cohort studies. Lancet 2009;373:1352–63.

39. Bell SK, Little SJ, Rosenberg ES. Clinical management of acute HIV infection: best practice remains unknown. J Infect Dis 2010;202(Suppl 2):S278–88.

40. Moir S, Buckner CM, Ho J, et al. B cells in early and chronic HIV infection: evidence for preservation of immune function associated with early initiation of antiretroviral therapy. Blood 2010;116:5571–9.

41. Fidler S, Fox J, Touloumi G, et al. Slower CD4 cell decline following cessation of a 3 month course of HAART in primary HIV infection: findings from an observational cohort. AIDS 2007;21:1283–91.

42. Laeyendecker O, Redd AD, Lutalo T, et al. Frequency of long-term nonprogressors in HIV-1 seroconverters from Rakai Uganda. J Acquir Immune Defic Syndr 2009;52:316–9.

43. Grabar S, Selinger-Leneman H, Abgrall S, et al. Prevalence and comparative characteristics of long-term nonprogressors and HIV controller patients in the French Hospital Database on HIV. AIDS 2009;23:1163–9.

44. Panel on Antiretroviral Guidelines for Adults and Adolescents. Guidelines for the use of antiretroviral agents in HIV-1-infected adults and adolescents. Washington, DC: Department of Health and Human Services; 2013. 10-30-2013.

45. Thompson MA, Aberg JA, Hoy JF, et al. Antiretroviral treatment of adult HIV infection: 2012 recommendations of the International Antiviral Society-USA panel. JAMA 2012;308:387–402.

46. Lundgren JD, Clumeck N, Rockstroh J. Guidelines version 7.0. Brussels (Belgium): European AIDS Clinical Society; 2013.

47. Williams I, Churchill D, Anderson J, et al. British HIV Association guidelines for the treatment of HIV-1-positive adults with antiretroviral therapy 2012 (Updated November 2013. All changed text is cast in yellow highlight.). HIV Med 2014; 15(Suppl 1):1–85.

48. HIV/AIDS Programme. Consolidated guidelines on the use of antiretroviral drugs for treating and preventing HIV infection: recommendations for a public health approach. Geneva (Switzerland): World Health Organization; 2013.

49. Gallant JE, Mehta SH, Sugarman J. Universal antiretroviral therapy for HIV infection: should US treatment guidelines be applied to resource-limited settings? Clin Infect Dis 2013;57:884–7.

50. Chang LW, Serwadda D, Quinn TC, et al. Combination implementation for HIV prevention: moving from clinical trial evidence to population-level effects. Lancet Infect Dis 2013;13:65–76.

51. Brenner BG, Roger M, Routy JP, et al. High rates of forward transmission events after acute/early HIV-1 infection. J Infect Dis 2007;195:951–9.

52. Cohen MS, Shaw GM, McMichael AJ, et al. Acute HIV-1 Infection. N Engl J Med 2011;364:1943–54.

53. Brown AE, Gill ON, Delpech VC. HIV treatment as prevention among men who have sex with men in the UK: is transmission controlled by universal access to HIV treatment and care? HIV Med 2013;14:563–70.

54. Koblin BA, Mayer KH, Eshleman SH, et al. Correlates of HIV acquisition in a cohort of Black men who have sex with men in the United States: HIV prevention trials network (HPTN) 061. PLoS One 2013;8:e70413.

55. Shisana O, Rehle T, Simbayi L, et al. South African national HIV prevalence, incidence, behaviour and communication survey 2008. Cape Town (South Africa): HSRC Press; 2009.

56. Ministry of Health and Social Welfare. Lesotho demographic and health survey 2009. Calverton (MD): ICF Macro; 2010.

57. Moyer VA. Screening for HIV: U.S. Preventive Services Task Force recommendation statement. Ann Intern Med 2013;159:51–60.

58. Branson BM, Handsfield HH, Lampe MA, et al. Revised recommendations for HIV testing of adults, adolescents, and pregnant women in health-care settings. MMWR Recomm Rep 2006;55:1–17.

59. Rosen S, Fox MP. Retention in HIV care between testing and treatment in sub-Saharan Africa: a systematic review. PLoS Med 2011;8:e1001056.

60. Gardner EM, McLees MP, Steiner JF, et al. The spectrum of engagement in HIV care and its relevance to test-and-treat strategies for prevention of HIV infection. Clin Infect Dis 2011;52:793–800.

61. Thompson MA, Mugavero MJ, Amico KR, et al. Guidelines for improving entry into and retention in care and antiretroviral adherence for persons with HIV: evidence-based recommendations from an International Association of Physicians in AIDS Care panel. Ann Intern Med 2012;156:817–33 W.

62. Gupta RK, Wainberg MA, Brun-Vezinet F, et al. Oral antiretroviral drugs as public health tools for HIV prevention: global implications for adherence, drug resistance, and the success of HIV treatment programs. J Infect Dis 2013; 207(Suppl 2):S101–6.

Pre-exposure Prophylaxis for Human Immunodeficiency Virus
The Past, Present, and Future

Amanda D. Castel, MD, MPH*, Manya Magnus, PhD, MPH,
Alan E. Greenberg, MD, MPH

KEYWORDS

- Pre-exposure prophylaxis • Implementation • Adherence • HIV prevention
- Biomedical intervention

KEY POINTS

- Our knowledge of pre-exposure prophylaxis (PrEP) as a means to prevent human immunodeficiency virus (HIV) acquisition has increased greatly over the decade.
- Evidence from clinical trials conducted among multiple high-risk populations suggests that oral PrEP, if adhered to, can be effective in reducing the risk of HIV acquisition among HIV-uninfected individuals.
- The key issues with PrEP use that have arisen as a result of these trials warranting further research include adherence, risk of drug resistance, and behavioral disinhibition.
- Studies further informing PrEP utilization are ongoing to address issues such as alternate dosing strategies and delivery methods, long-term side effects, and effectiveness in real-world settings.
- PrEP implementation is underway; future studies and activities will need to focus on optimizing PrEP regimens and adherence, increasing education and uptake among high-risk populations and providers, and establishing systems to monitor and evaluate PrEP use.

INTRODUCTION

Human immunodeficiency virus (HIV) prevention research has rapidly advanced over the last decade, with several large-scale research studies demonstrating that antiretrovirals (ARVs) can be used not only for the prevention of mother-to-child transmission, post-exposure prophylaxis, and treatment as prevention (TasP) but also for

Department of Epidemiology and Biostatistics, Milken Institute School of Public Health, The George Washington University, 950 New Hampshire Avenue, Northwest, 5th Floor, Washington, DC 20052, USA
* Corresponding author.
E-mail address: acastel@gwu.edu

Infect Dis Clin N Am 28 (2014) 563–583
http://dx.doi.org/10.1016/j.idc.2014.08.001
0891-5520/14/$ – see front matter © 2014 Elsevier Inc. All rights reserved.

id.theclinics.com

pre-exposure prophylaxis (PrEP). PrEP for HIV prevention involves the use of ARV medications, optimally delivered in concert with risk-reduction counseling and behavioral interventions, such as condom provision and use, to prevent HIV infection among those who are HIV uninfected but at high risk for infection. PrEP entails having an HIV-uninfected individual take ARVs orally or topically (either vaginally or rectally) to prevent sexual or parenteral infection with HIV.[1,2]

The concept of PrEP is not new and has been used as a prevention method for a variety of illnesses, including prevention against rabies[3] and malaria[4] among those traveling to endemic areas. PrEP was considered as a strategy to reduce the number of new HIV infections given the continued high HIV incidence rates both nationally and globally. Globally, an estimated 2.5 million new infections occur every year[5]; in the United States, there are an estimated 50,000 new infections annually.[6] Without an effective HIV vaccine on the horizon, the need for high-impact HIV prevention tools is essential. These tools include interventions such as TasP for HIV-infected individuals; routine HIV testing and linkage to care; and biomedical interventions, such as male circumcision.[7]

Further research into PrEP will add to the toolbox of HIV prevention methods.

This article describes the prior research that informs our current understanding of PrEP, summarizes ongoing research in the area, and highlights key issues that must be addressed in order to optimize the use of this HIV prevention tool.

THE PAST: DEVELOPMENT OF PRE-EXPOSURE PROPHYLAXIS AS AN HIV PREVENTION INTERVENTION
Prior Evidence of Use of Antiretrovirals for Prevention

Proof of concept for the use of PrEP to prevent HIV infection stems from research conducted in both animals and humans. The use of PrEP and postexposure prophylaxis to prevent mother-to-child transmission of HIV has been proven to reduce the risk of transmission by as much as 99%.[8–10] Similarly, the use of postexposure prophylaxis in situations in which a person has had a high-risk sexual or parenteral exposure, or a high-risk occupational exposure, has been shown to be effective with an 81% reduction in transmission.[11] This proof of concept led to the first HIV PrEP trials using animal models.

Animal Trials

The biological plausibility of using ARVs as PrEP for HIV prevention was first examined using animal models as early as 1995. These animal studies also assisted in understanding issues regarding which drugs would be efficacious, drug delivery, and dosing. Among the many ARVs available, tenofovir disoproxil fumarate (TDF), a nucleoside reverse transcriptase inhibitor, has been widely studied for use as both oral and vaginal PrEP. This ARV is generally well-tolerated in HIV-infected persons and has minimal side effects.[12] The combination of tenofovir (TDF) and emtricitabine (FTC) (Truvada) has also been extensively studied for use with PrEP and has been used in many of the animal and clinical trials conducted to date.

The first few nonhuman primate studies assessed the efficacy of injectable TDF for PrEP. In 1995, Tsai and colleagues[13] published data that found that 4 weeks of daily injections of TDF starting 48 hours before, 4 hours after, or 24 hours after intravenous simian immunodeficiency virus (SIV) challenge resulted in 100% protection in macaques. In 1998, Van Rompay and colleagues[14] also concluded that 2 injectable doses of TDF 4 hours before and 20 hours after oral SIV challenge resulted in 100% protection among newborn macaques.

Although the initial injectable PrEP animal studies found 100% protection, early studies examining daily oral dosing with TDF followed by oral or rectal exposure did not. A series of studies found either no or partial efficacy after oral exposure[15,16] or delayed infections after rectal exposure.[17] Not until 2008 did studies looking at FTC in combination with oral TDF begin to show efficacy in reducing the risk of infection. In 2008 and 2010, studies were published that demonstrated that daily oral and intermittent oral PrEP with FTC and TDF/FTC was efficacious, providing either partial or complete protection.[18–20] These findings demonstrated not only that TDF/FTC was able to provide a high level of protection but also that TDF/FTC could be used in lieu of TDF for PrEP, thereby lowering the risk of potential drug resistance in the event of seroconversion.[19] Finally, studies of vaginal delivery of 1% TDF gel applied topically before exposure were also shown to be fully protective.[21]

Hence, these animal studies provided evidence that either TDF or and TDF/FTC could be used to prevent infection; given through injections; taken orally either daily or intermittently; and, most importantly, were efficacious in providing protection from oral, rectal, and vaginal exposure.

Randomized Clinical Trials Among Humans

These nonhuman primate study findings coupled with other confirmatory animal studies[22] supported the introduction of clinical trials of PrEP among humans. Since 2011, results from phase I, II, and III clinical trials have focused on different medications, delivery methods, and high-risk populations. Many of these studies have confirmed the efficacy of ARVs for HIV prevention among high-risk populations, including men who have sex with men (MSM), high-risk heterosexual men and women, serodiscordant couples, and most recently among injection drug users (IDUs) (**Table 1**).[23–28]

Following safety evidence provided by phase I and phase II studies of PrEP among HIV-uninfected persons using TDF and TDF/FTC,[22,29] several landmark studies demonstrated the efficacy of PrEP in reducing HIV transmission. Five key studies have paved the way for future use of PrEP: the Center for AIDS Program of Research in South Africa (CAPRISA) 004, Pre-exposure Prophylaxis Initiative (iPrEx) trial, TDF2, Partners PrEP, and the Bangkok Tenofovir study. The CAPRISA 004 trial sought to assess the safety and efficacy of using a 1% vaginal gel formulation of TDF among heterosexual women in Africa.[23] Participants used the gel both before and after coitus. After 30 months of follow-up, it was determined that the use of the TDF gel reduced the risk of infection by 39% when compared with the placebo arm. Subsequent as-treated analyses found that among women taking greater than 80% of doses, the efficacy increased to 54%, although these post hoc analyses should be interpreted cautiously. Thus, the CAPRISA study was able to confirm that a vaginal gel for PrEP could be used safely and effectively by women for HIV prevention.

The iPrEx trial was one of the first to examine the efficacy of daily oral TDF/FTC use for PrEP among MSM and among transgender women compared with placebo. Approximately 2500 participants were enrolled from multiple countries and followed for a median of 21 months. In as-treated analyses, daily oral TDF/FTC was found to reduce the risk of infection by 44% among participants in the TDF/FTC arm, with further as-treated analyses indicating that among those taking pills on 90% or more of days, the efficacy increased to 73% and was more than 90% in those with detectable drug levels.[26]

The TDF2 study, conducted in Botswana, sought to assess the efficacy of oral TDF/FTC as PrEP among heterosexual men and women. Participants were randomized to receive either daily oral TDF/FTC or placebo. Taking daily TDF/FTC reduced the risk of

Table 1
Summary of completed PrEP trials

Study Name	Study Start Date	Target Population and Sample Size	Study Locations	Study Regimen	Overall Efficacy (%) (95% CI)	Efficacy Among Adherent Population[a] (%)
Bangkok Tenofovir Study	2005	IDUs (N = 2413)	Thailand	Oral TDF	49 (10–72)	74
CAPRISIA	2007	Heterosexual women (N = 889)	South Africa	Vaginal TFV	39 (6–60)	54
TDF2	2007	Heterosexual men and women (N = 1219)	Botswana	Oral TDF/FTC	62 (22–83)	78
iPrEx	2007	MSM and transgender women (N = 2499)	Brazil, Ecuador, Peru, South Africa, Thailand, United States	Oral TDF/FTC	44 (15–63)	73–90
Partners PrEP	2008	Serodiscordant heterosexual couples (N = 4758)	Kenya, Uganda	Oral TDF Oral TDF/FTC	TDF: 67 (44–81) TDF/FTC: 75 (55–87)	86–90
FEM-PrEP	2009	Heterosexual women (N = 2120)	Kenya, South Africa, Tanzania	Oral TDF/FTC	6 (−52 to 41)	18–25
VOICE	2009	Heterosexual women (N = 5029)	Uganda, South Africa, Zimbabwe	Oral TDF Oral TDF/FTC	TFV: 15 (−20 to 40) TDF: −49 (−129 to 3) TDF/FTC: −4 (−49 to 27)	Study stopped for futility

Abbreviations: CAPRISIA, Center for AIDS Program of Research in South Africa; CI, confidence interval; iPrEx, Pre-exposure Prophylaxis Initiative; TFV, 1% tenofovir vaginal gel; VOICE, Vaginal and Oral Interventions to Control the Epidemic.
[a] Adherence was determined using different outcomes according to each study protocol.

HIV infection by 62% and increased to 78% among those confirmed to have received drug in the prior 30 days.[24] When one previously undiagnosed HIV-infected participant receiving TDF/FTC developed drug resistance, the TDF2 study results highlighted the important potential for drug resistance among seroconverters and the need to identify these people as early in their infections as possible.

The Partners PrEP study was conducted in Kenya and Uganda among HIV-1 sero-discordant couples. Participants were randomized to one of three study arms: daily oral TDF, daily oral TDF/FTC, or matching placebo.[27] Final analysis showed a 67% reduction in the risk of HIV transmission among the TDF arm and a 75% reduction among the TDF/FTC arm with no issues regarding safety or tolerability.[27] When assessing efficacy among those with detectable TDF drug levels, efficacy was 86% and 90% among the TDF and TDF/FTC arms, respectively.[30]

Finally, the Bangkok Tenofovir study in Thailand was the only study to date to evaluate the use of PrEP among IDUs.[31] A unique feature of this study was that study participants received oral TDF or placebo via directly observed therapy, rather than independently. Primary analysis found a 49% reduction in HIV infection among the participants receiving TDF compared with a 74% reduction among those observed while taking their medications who had detectable TDF drug levels.[25]

Although these landmark studies support the efficacy of oral PrEP among MSM, heterosexuals, men, women, and IDUs, as well as vaginal PrEP among women, 2 other large PrEP studies have shown little to no efficacy among women. The Vaginal and Oral Interventions to Control the Epidemic (VOICE) study, which enrolled women living in Southern Africa, randomized women into one of 5 study arms. These arms included daily vaginal gel with and without TDF, daily oral TDF, daily oral TDF/FTC, and daily matching oral placebo. Initial analysis found that neither the daily oral nor the vaginal TDF arms reduced the risk of HIV infection, and final analyses found that the daily oral TDF/FTC arm was also not efficacious in reducing the participants' risk of HIV infection.[32] Since publication of these findings, additional analyses determined that adherence, as measured by product use, was very low among study participants and may have explained these disparate results.

Similar to the VOICE trial findings, the FEM-PrEP study sought to assess the efficacy of PrEP among African heterosexual women, randomizing participants to receive either daily oral TDF/FTC or placebo.[28] The study was terminated prematurely after interim analyses found similar rates of HIV infection among both study arms. Poor adherence, as in the VOICE trial, was thought to explain the lack of efficacy, as low levels of plasma TDF were measured among women who became infected during the study period.[33] These studies underscore the important role of adherence in both researching and implementing PrEP.

Implementation of Pre-exposure Prophylaxis

With the results from most of the phase III trials showing efficacy, in July 2012, the US Food and Drug Administration (FDA) approved licensure of TDF/FTC for daily oral use as PrEP among HIV-uninfected persons at high-risk for infection.[34] Although other ARVs have been evaluated for use as for PrEP, TDF/FTC is currently the only approved ARV with this indicated use. This instance was the first time that an ARV for HIV has been approved for both prevention in uninfected persons and for treatment of HIV. In response to the availability of this new biomedical prevention intervention, the US Centers for Disease Control and Prevention has issued guidance documents for clinicians considering prescribing PrEP to MSM, IDUs, and heterosexuals at high risk for HIV.[35–38] The World Health Organization has also issued guidance for the use of PrEP among serodiscordant couples, MSM, and transgender women who have sex with men.[39]

Multiple demonstration projects are underway to assist in the scale-up of PrEP as an HIV prevention method in the United States and in Africa; these include open access programs to support PrEP use provided by the pharmaceutical company that makes Truvada,[40] HPTN 073,[41] and various locally administered agency-based programs.[42]

Lessons Learned from the Past

Safety
All of the aforementioned studies have shown acceptable levels of safety and tolerability. Most common short-term side effects reported in these studies have included nausea, headaches, and weight loss[24,26–28]; however, monitoring for longer-term side effects, such as hepatic toxicity, kidney toxicity, and bone density loss, will need to be conducted.

Resistance
Poor adherence when using ARVs for PrEP can increase one's risk of infection with resistant strains if a person seroconverts and can subsequently limit one's future treatment options.[43] Reassuringly, when participants on the studies referenced seroconverted, drug resistance among incident cases was relatively rare. As few as none and as many as 3 participants were reported to develop resistance,[12,24,26,27,44] usually to FTC, although it is important to remember that these studies were not statistically powered to assess the development of resistance.

Adherence
Adherence has often been described as the Achilles heel of PrEP, with both the VOICE and FEM-PrEP studies emphasizing the essential role that adherence plays in ensuring the efficacy of using ARVs for PrEP.[45] As discussed, among five key PrEP clinical trials, efficacy was notably higher among the more adherent participants when compared to the overall study population.[24,26–28,46–49] For example, in iPrEX, the overall efficacy was 44%; but among those with detectable drug, the efficacy increased to 92%.[26] Similarly, the FEM-PrEP study showed that the overall efficacy was a mere 6%, possibly because of low adherence.[28]

For many of these studies, post hoc, as-treated analyses should be interpreted cautiously, as they violate assumptions of intention-to-treat analysis and, thus, may reflect underlying differences between persons who adhere to medications and those who do not, rather than the intrinsic benefits of the medication itself. Therefore, going forward, when prescribing PrEP, education, assessment of a patient's ability to adhere to treatment, as well as follow-up safety monitoring visits will be critical in reducing the risk of HIV acquisition and development of resistant infection. Studies, described hereafter, are underway to further study interventions to increase adherence among PrEP users.

Behavioral disinhibition
With the availability and use of PrEP, concerns have been raised regarding behavioral disinhibition/risk compensation (eg, having more high-risk sex partners or engaging in more unprotected and higher-risk sex acts because one is taking PrEP).[50,51] PrEP is a part of a combination prevention method; therefore, all persons receiving it through clinical trials also receive risk-reduction counseling and are encouraged to use condoms. None of the studies described earlier have observed any significant behavioral disinhibition, yet this may present a real concern among persons using PrEP in nonclinical trial settings. Adherence to PrEP regimens needs to be a focus area as PrEP is scaled up in community settings; ensuring adequate complementary behavioral education and services alongside PrEP delivery will also be critical.

THE PRESENT: ASSESSMENT OF NEW REGIMENS, DELIVERY MECHANISMS, AND FEASIBILITY

The issues presented in the previous section regarding PrEP safety, the development of viral resistance among seroconverters, adherence, and behavioral disinhibition inform many of the studies currently in progress. Even as PrEP is rapidly translated into practice, research continues to further our knowledge of this biomedical prevention strategy.[52–54] Current studies are designed to identify prevention regimens more effective than TDF/FTC with less viral resistance potential as well as to develop new modes of administration that overcome barriers to adherence.[55–65] Further, several open-label demonstration projects are being conducted that aim to characterize the correlates of PrEP uptake in key affected populations.[41,42] This section describes examples of ongoing research that leverage past successes of PrEP and strive to expand opportunities for PrEP use into the future.

New Pre-exposure Prophylaxis Regimens

Given the use of TDF/FTC in many first-line regimens for HIV-infected persons, one key concern is identification of a PrEP agent for which the development of resistance among seroconverters, however few there are, would have less impact. Maraviroc (MVC) was FDA approved in 2007 as the treatment of HIV following demonstration of virologic suppression among HIV-infected persons.[66] This CCR5 antagonist has been used safely among this population and found to have an acceptable safety profile, and it is currently not a first-line treatment regimen.[54,66–68] MVC was considered a potential agent for use as PrEP because of its biological mechanism of action. Unlike TDF and FTC, MVC surrounds the CCR5 coreceptor, allowing MVC to interrupt viral binding early in the HIV lifecycle. Early primate studies demonstrated that MVC prevented simian HIV (SHIV) infection against rectal HIV-1 challenges as well as when it was used as a microbicide agent against vaginal challenges, although more recent studies of MVC among macaques indicated no HIV prevention activity against rectal SHIV compared with controls, even in the presence of adequate blood levels.[19,67,69–71] Other studies have shown protection against vaginal introduction of SHIV in macaques using MVC,[72–74] though results using intravaginal rings (IVR) among primates have been mixed.[75,76] These characteristics in combination with its ability to concentrate high levels of drug in the cervicovaginal and rectal tissues relative to plasma levels make MVC a potentially powerful PrEP agent to explore in humans. MVC has been studied among 450 HIV-uninfected persons with rheumatoid arthritis,[77] but this was for short-term (12 weeks) use only and not among a population identified as at high risk for HIV. However, its favorable safety results contributed to another ongoing clinical trial in the United States. In 2011, the National Institutes of Health–funded HIV Prevention Trials Network (HPTN) launched HPTN 069, a phase II, randomized, placebo-controlled, double-blinded, multisite study of MVC as PrEP, comparing 3 arms: MVC versus MVC+TDF versus MVC+FTC versus TDF+FTC (**Table 2**). This study, initially open only to men and transgender women (male at birth), expanded eligibility in 2013 to include biologically born women. Data from HPTN 069, will characterize the safety and tolerability of MVC among an HIV-uninfected population at an elevated risk for HIV and determine whether this potentially promising PrEP agent will move forward to phase III efficacy trials.[68]

Novel Formulations

In addition to the search for additional PrEP agents that are effective, better tolerated, and with low potential to develop resistance, as well as not competing with first-line

Table 2
New PrEP agents under study in 2014

Agent	Description of Drug	Methods of Delivery Under Study
Maraviroc	CCR5 antagonist	Oral; vaginal ring
Dapivirine	Non-nucleoside reverse transcriptase inhibitor	Vaginal ring
GSK1265744/LA	Integrase strand-inhibitor; long-acting analogue to dolutegravir	Oral; injectable (long acting)
TMC-278/LA	Long-acting formulation of rilpivirine	Oral; injectable (long acting)

treatment regimens as does TDF/FTC, a key goal among current research is the development of formulations to overcome barriers to adherence. As described earlier, all of the studies evaluating PrEP as prevention against sexual HIV acquisition,[24,27,28,49] and even the directly observed therapy administration to IDU,[25,46] were undermined by poor adherence. As a result, new long-acting formulations that are either injectable or, for women, used as IVR hold promise to overcome barriers to PrEP adherence. Multiple products showing promise in this regard are currently in the pipeline (see **Table 2**). For example, the recently FDA-approved integrase strand-inhibitor dolutegravir (Tivicay) has been shown to be an effective treatment among both ARV-experienced and ARV–naïve HIV-infected patients.[55–57,59–64] With its favorable safety profile and characteristics amenable to formulation as a long-acting agent (eg, potency, solubility, and melting point), this long-acting analogue to dolutegravir, GSK1265744LA, is potentially seen as an ideal candidate for long-acting PrEP, either as a monthly or a quarterly injection.[55–57,59–64] In addition to its physical properties, GSK1265744LA has been shown to be highly effective as PrEP when tested among macaques in a recent trial of SHIV prevention following rectal challenge.[55,56] A phase IIb randomized trial of the safety and tolerability of this agent is expected to begin among low-risk men and women in 2014 in 2 separate complementary studies in the United States, South America, and sub-Saharan Africa.

Another long-acting agent, TMC-278LA, is the long-acting formulation of (marketed as Edurant alone and together with TDF/FTC in Complera) a non-nucleoside reverse transcriptase inhibitor approved for use in the United States by the FDA in 2011. This agent has similarly been shown to be safe, tolerable, and have a favorable profile for long-acting delivery.[57,58,62] This treatment has been used effectively among HIV-infected persons, including as the first-line treatment of treatment-naïve individuals.[62] Small-scale, phase I studies have shown TMC-278LA to be well tolerated when administered intramuscularly.[58,62,78,79] This agent, too, is slated to begin a phase IIb randomized trial of the safety and tolerability among low-risk men and women in 2014 in the United States and sub-Saharan Africa.[80] The availability of long-acting formulations, particularly those that need only be administered quarterly, will offer significant adherence benefits compared with daily use.

IVRs offer another formulation of PrEP that will be useful in overcoming adherence barriers for women. These flexible rings do not require insertion by a health care provider, as they can be inserted by women monthly.[53,54,79] Benefits of the ring when compared with a long-acting injectable include the potential for simultaneous administration of PrEP and hormonal contraceptive; the ability to remove the ring in the event of changing HIV risk profiles; and, in the event of allergic reaction or side effect, increased ability to halt the dosing.[81] Previous studies have indicated efficacy at preventing vaginal SHIV infection after challenge with dapivirine, though the IVR with MVC has been less effective in primate trials.[81]

Open-Label Investigations

Perhaps as critical to the PrEP conversation as are new formulations is the question of scale-up. PrEP is one of the first available biomedical HIV prevention interventions; as such, few data exist regarding optimal methods of implementation among those at highest risk of HIV. Simply the availability of PrEP does not ensure uptake, particularly among persons at the highest risk of HIV who may not have access to health care or costly prescriptions.[82–88] In addition to ongoing clinical trials of new and currently approved PrEP agents described earlier, investigations are being conducted to characterize the way PrEP is disseminated outside of the ideal clinical trials environment.

Several investigations of open-label PrEP are currently ongoing in the United States. These investigations include iPrEx open label extension (OLE), the optional, open-label follow-on study to the iPrEx study[89]; HPTN 073, offering open-label TDF/FTC to black MSM in concert with a client-centered case management intervention[41]; and local demonstration sites exploring provision of PrEP, largely in urban centers.[90–92] These studies generally explore correlates of PrEP uptake, adherence behavior, sexual and other HIV-related risk behavior while taking PrEP, and myriad characteristics that will eventually inform wider distribution of PrEP. Outside of research trials and demonstration sites, there are few ways to obtain PrEP free of charge, but there are pharmaceutical company-sponsored assistance programs[40] and copay programs for PrEP[93] available. In addition, private insurance as well as that through the Affordable Care Act[1] will pay for or subsidize PrEP prescriptions with varying degrees of preauthorization and documentation. Despite these offerings, the number of PrEP prescriptions in the United States since FDA approval of TDF/FTC remains quite low.[94,95]

THE FUTURE: PRE-EXPOSURE PROPHYLAXIS IMPLEMENTATION

In the previous section, the authors provided an overview of the current research efforts to assess new PrEP regimens, novel PrEP formulations, and the feasibility of scaling up PrEP in high-risk populations in nonclinical trials settings. In this section, the authors address 4 areas that will need to be considered when strategizing about the scale-up of PrEP on a population-wide basis: (1) optimization of PrEP regimens, (2) delivery of PrEP, (3) engagement of high-risk populations; and (4) guidelines, goals and monitoring, and evaluation.

Optimization of Pre-exposure Prophylaxis Regimens

The numerous clinical trials summarized earlier clearly indicate that even in the research setting, a substantial proportion of persons who might benefit from PrEP are unable or unwilling to adhere to a daily oral regimen. Similar to other biomedical prevention behaviors, such as oral contraceptives[96] or preventive vaccines,[4,97] adherence to daily regimens or to prevention guidelines involve the complex interplay between knowledge, attitudes, and behavior. Taking daily medication to prevent HIV acquisition requires numerous behavioral steps. Perception of self-risk must be sufficient to take a pill daily, even if behavioral risks are not present each day, because of the need to maintain adequate blood levels.[26] An individual's assessment that the medication is worth taking despite the side effects, as well as change in acceptance of medication-related risks over time because of the unknown long-term impacts of taking PrEP,[45,47,98] may result in varying adherence over the life cycle. Overcoming concerns about stigma if possession of the medications alone discloses high-risk behavior or the concern that having ARVs makes others think that patients are HIV infected are also barriers to adherence.[48,99] Finally, even with appropriate knowledge, self-risk assessment, and the means to obtain and take the medication, daily adherence can be a struggle[45–48]; many people do not adhere, even with no frank reasons for nonadherence.

Additionally, the impact of PrEP regimens on the development of ARV resistance in persons who become HIV infected while taking PrEP will also need to be considered. Monitoring provided by a clinical trial environment differs substantially from a community-based care approach. For example, study participants in trials are generally tested for HIV monthly or every 8 weeks, whereas in real-world settings, testing is recommended every 3 months. Persons on PrEP who do seroconvert are at an increased risk of resistance the longer the duration of treatment on PrEP continues after infection because of the difference in treatment regimens and doses prescribed for infection versus prevention. Reconciling clinical trials' standards with care delivery in real-world settings with regard to appropriate monitoring will be an important area of focus as PrEP is made more widely available.

Concurrently, the safety of longer-term PrEP administration will need to be considered, as current research studies have followed those taking PrEP for only 2 to 3 years. The IPrEx OLE study is continuing to follow PrEP users taking TDF/FTC and will soon be able to provide information on longer-term safety and efficacy; similarly long-term follow-up studies both within and outside of clinical trial settings will need to be conducted as new, longer-acting PrEP regimens are developed.

Lastly, the targeting of PrEP use during periods of risk will continue to emerge as an important issue. PrEP scale-up has been compared with that of birth control,[96] in that women may elect to use oral or injectable birth control methods during periods of time when they do not desire to get pregnant. Similarly, persons at risk for HIV may elect to use PrEP for short periods of time during high-risk activity (eg, multiple sexual partners), for longer periods of time (eg, serodiscordant relationships), or may cycle on and off PrEP. This usage is also similar to models such as malaria prophylaxis, which can be used for a short duration (travel to malaria-endemic areas) or for longer durations (eg, living in malaria-endemic areas).[100]

Delivery of Pre-exposure Prophylaxis

Challenges to delivery and scale-up of PrEP have been identified, largely because of the issues around payment coverage for the drugs,[101] uncertainties of prescribing among many community-based noninfectious disease physicians (where most HIV-uninfected persons are seen for care),[102,103] minimal access to studies or free demonstration projects,[42] and challenges in engaging and treating high-risk populations who are likely most in need of the prevention intervention that PrEP represents.[82,104,105] First, there are issues regarding which clinical providers will prescribe PrEP and monitor its use by patients. Most HIV-uninfected persons who will be eligible for PrEP are seen by community-based noninfectious disease physicians who may be unaware of PrEP guidelines, feel uncomfortable discussing sexual or drug use behavior with patients, and do not have substantial experience prescribing ARVs.[102,106–108] Alternatively, PrEP could be delivered by infectious disease specialists with expertise in HIV and ARVs; but their capacity and willingness to provide PrEP for large numbers of HIV-uninfected persons may vary by provider. Another challenge presaged by the minimal availability of free or discounted PrEP is the transition into community-based access following the discontinuation of subsidized PrEP. Future programs will need to overcome this challenge and prospectively identify procedures for roll-off from clinical trials and open-label demonstration projects once these programs end.

Additionally, there are important cost, insurance coverage, and access considerations that will also need to be considered if PrEP is to be implemented on a wider basis given the high cost of ARVs. Although cost-effectiveness studies have indicated that PrEP is cost-effective in areas with high HIV prevalence, generalized epidemics, and among high-risk populations,[101,109–114] the longer-term costs of HIV testing and monitoring will also need to be considered.[101] At present in the United States, financial coverage for PrEP depends on one's health insurance or willingness to self-pay; it will be important to monitor the impact of the Affordable Care Act on coverage for PrEP as well as changing private insurance paradigms for coverage of PrEP. Currently, there is limited access to PrEP through research studies and demonstration projects,[42] and Gilead Sciences, which manufactures Truvada, has developed a patient assistance program to assist patients who seek PrEP but do not have insurance coverage.[40]

Globally, there are country-specific issues related to PrEP access, including payment options and the development of national PrEP guidelines. In addition, issues related to resource allocation have been raised regarding supporting PrEP implementation both domestically and globally when there are still many untreated HIV-infected persons in need of ARV therapy.[115] The World Health Organization has issued guidance that, for serodiscordant couples when the HIV-infected partner may not yet be eligible for ARV treatment as per country guidelines, PrEP can be considered for the uninfected partner for 6 months as a bridge to treatment.[39] Moreover, the use of TasP is now established as an important component of HIV prevention programs both domestically and globally, which could potentially modulate enthusiasm for directing limited resources toward PrEP.

Engagement of High-Risk Populations

Despite the efficacy of PrEP in reducing the individual risk of HIV acquisition, many potential users in high-risk populations remain unaware of the potential benefits of PrEP and how to access this intervention.[116,117] Educational initiatives are being developed for persons at high HIV risk who may benefit from PrEP, including mobile phone applications, Web sites to assess one's risk for HIV, adherence interventions,[118] and the issuance of PrEP guidance documents for interested participants and providers by state health departments.[119,120]

Stigma remains a considerable barrier to PrEP provision, in the context of prescribing and using PrEP as well as adherence. Because ARV use for prevention and treatment can easily be confused, uninfected persons may be reluctant to use PrEP as friends and family members may think they are HIV infected.[45] In addition, the use of PrEP also signals high-risk sexual or drug use behavior and may suggest gay or bisexual orientation among men, drug use in men and women, and nonmonogamy in couples. This problem may be obviated by clinic-based injections when long-acting formulations become available, but daily regimens and IVRs will not eliminate these factors. For oral PrEP, changes in packaging that distinguish the use of PrEP for prevention from treatment may ultimately facilitate acceptance of and adherence to PrEP, much as oral contraceptives benefit from packaging that enables daily adherence. Risk compensation is a frequent issue that emerges in discussions of PrEP scale-up, as the prevention benefits of PrEP as a biomedical intervention can be mitigated by behavioral factors, such as an increase in numbers of sexual partners or a decrease in condom use.[121]

Consideration of issues related to gender will also be important as PrEP use becomes more widespread to ensure that this prevention modality meets the needs of women. In the United States, women have been underrepresented in PrEP studies and demonstration projects, although women are included in the Centers for Disease Control and Prevention's PrEP guidelines and the FDA approval of TDF/FTC for PrEP.[34,36] Globally, women have been well represented in PrEP trials; but caution will be required translating lessons learned outside of the United States to women in the United States, just as the converse is true for MSM. The complex relationship for women regarding PrEP in the context of pregnancy prevention, pregnancy, and desired family building will also necessitate further exploration.[122,123]

Guidelines, Goals and Monitoring, and Evaluation

The use of oral PrEP for individuals at high risk of HIV infection has been shown to be a safe and effective HIV prevention intervention. Scaling the use of PrEP to a population-based level,[124] however, will be an ongoing public health challenge that will require awareness of numerous issues, several of which are described earlier. Moving forward, a higher degree of granularity and regular updating of PrEP guidelines will be needed as new ARVs are demonstrated to be safe and effective for PrEP use; longer-acting PrEP formulations become available; different patterns of intermittent PrEP use are evaluated; PrEP uptake increases in various high-risk populations; and the role of PrEP is further evaluated in discordant couples in which the HIV-infected partner is virologically suppressed on ARVs. For example, more data will be needed with regard to how to use PrEP over the life cycle: as behavioral risk profiles change, guidelines for how PrEP use should change will be necessary. Similarly, for discordant couples in which the HIV-infected partner is adherent to ARV and virologically suppressed, more data will be needed to discern whether the addition of PrEP is cost-effective and warrants added medication risks to the uninfected partner. Moreover, although it may be premature at present, the development of local, regional, and global quantifiable goals for PrEP use will be useful to promote the scale-up of PrEP use to impactful levels, especially if long-acting PrEP formulations become available. Lastly, as PrEP use becomes more widespread,[125] innovative monitoring and evaluation systems will need to be developed for PrEP uptake, adherence, ARV resistance, safety, and efficacy. As PrEP becomes more widely available and people become more aware about its benefits, research inquiries into these more nuanced facets of PrEP deserve exploration.

SUMMARY

In the past decade, enormous progress has been made in the development of PrEP as an HIV prevention intervention, with the safety and efficacy of PrEP now demonstrated in MSM, IDUs, and heterosexuals. Current research is ongoing to assess new PrEP ARV regimens, alternative and long-acting PrEP delivery mechanisms, and the feasibility of implementing PrEP in high-risk populations. In the years ahead, the HIV prevention field will continue to address several critical issues, including the optimization of PrEP regimens, how best to support the delivery of PrEP on a population-level scale, engagement of high-risk populations, the updating of PrEP guidelines, and the establishment of PrEP-related goals and monitoring and evaluation systems.

REFERENCES

1. AIDS.Gov. Preexposure prophylaxis (PrEP). 2013. Available at: http://aids.gov/hiv-aids-basics/prevention/reduce-your-risk/pre-exposure-prophylaxis/. Accessed April 2, 2014.
2. Centers for Disease Control and Prevention. Pre exposure prophylaxis: questions and answers. 2013. Available at: http://www.cdc.gov/hiv/prevention/research/prep/. Accessed April 2, 2014.
3. World Health Organization. International travel and health: rabies. Available at: http://www.who.int/ith/vaccines/rabies/en/. Accessed April 18, 2014.

4. Centers for Disease Control and Prevention. Infectious diseases related to travel: malaria. In: Arguin P, Tan K, editors. CDC Health Information for International Travel 2014. New York: Oxford University Press; 2014. Available at: http://wwwnc.cdc.gov/travel/yellowbook/2014/chapter-3-infectious-diseases-related-to-travel/malaria.

5. UNAIDS. Global report: UNAIDS report on the global AIDS epidemic 2013. 2013. Available at: http://www.unaids.org/en/resources/campaigns/globalreport2013/globalreport/. Accessed February 15, 2014.

6. Centers for Disease Control and Prevention. Estimated HIV incidence in the United States, 2007–2010. HIV Surveillance Supplemental Report 2012;17(4). Available at: http://www.cdc.gov/hiv/topics/surveillance/resources/reports/#supplemental. Accessed March 2, 2014.

7. Centers for Disease Control and Prevention. High-impact HIV prevention: CDC's approach to reducing HIV infections in the United States. 2013. Available at: http://www.cdc.gov/hiv/policies/hip.html. Accessed March 2, 2014.

8. Connor EM, Sperling RS, Gelber R, et al. Reduction of maternal-infant transmission of human immunodeficiency virus type 1 with zidovudine treatment. Pediatric AIDS Clinical Trials Group Protocol 076 Study Group. N Engl J Med 1994; 331(18):1173–80. http://dx.doi.org/10.1056/NEJM199411033311801.

9. Rates of mother-to-child transmission of HIV-1 in Africa, America, and Europe: results from 13 perinatal studies. The working group on mother-to-child transmission of HIV. J Acquir Immune Defic Syndr Hum Retrovirol 1995;8(5):506–10.

10. Siegfried N, van der Merwe L, Brocklehurst P, et al. Antiretrovirals for reducing the risk of mother-to-child transmission of HIV infection. Cochrane Database Syst Rev 2011;(7):CD003510. http://dx.doi.org/10.1002/14651858.CD003510.pub3.

11. Cardo DM, Culver DH, Ciesielski CA, et al. A case-control study of HIV seroconversion in health care workers after percutaneous exposure. Centers for Disease Control and Prevention Needlestick Surveillance Group. N Engl J Med 1997; 337(21):1485–90. http://dx.doi.org/10.1056/NEJM199711203372101.

12. Plosker GL. Emtricitabine/tenofovir disoproxil fumarate: a review of its use in HIV-1 pre-exposure prophylaxis. Drugs 2013;73(3):279–91. http://dx.doi.org/10.1007/s40265-013-0024-4.

13. Tsai CC, Follis KE, Sabo A, et al. Prevention of SIV infection in macaques by (R)-9-(2-phosphonylmethoxypropyl) adenine. Science 1995;270(5239):1197–9.

14. Van Rompay KK, Berardi CJ, Aguirre NL, et al. Two doses of PMPA protect newborn macaques against oral simian immunodeficiency virus infection. AIDS 1998;12(9):F79–83.

15. Van Rompay KK, Schmidt KA, Lawson JR, et al. Topical administration of low-dose tenofovir disoproxil fumarate to protect infant macaques against multiple oral exposures of low doses of simian immunodeficiency virus. J Infect Dis 2002;186(10):1508–13 pii:JID020627.

16. Van Rompay KK, Kearney BP, Sexton JJ, et al. Evaluation of oral tenofovir disoproxil fumarate and topical tenofovir GS-7340 to protect infant macaques against repeated oral challenges with virulent simian immunodeficiency virus. J Acquir Immune Defic Syndr 2006;43(1):6–14. http://dx.doi.org/10.1097/01.qai.0000224972.60339.7c.

17. Subbarao S, Otten RA, Ramos A, et al. Chemoprophylaxis with tenofovir disoproxil fumarate provided partial protection against infection with simian human immunodeficiency virus in macaques given multiple virus challenges. J Infect Dis 2006;194(7):904–11.

18. Garcia-Lerma JG, Cong ME, Mitchell J, et al. Intermittent prophylaxis with oral truvada protects macaques from rectal SHIV infection. Sci Transl Med 2010; 2(14):14ra4. http://dx.doi.org/10.1126/scitranslmed.3000391.

19. Garcia-Lerma JG, Otten RA, Qari SH, et al. Prevention of rectal SHIV transmission in macaques by daily or intermittent prophylaxis with emtricitabine and tenofovir. PLoS Med 2008;5(2):e28. http://dx.doi.org/10.1371/journal.pmed.0050028.

20. Cong ME, Youngpairoj AS, Zheng Q, et al. Protection against rectal transmission of an emtricitabine-resistant simian/human immunodeficiency virus SHIV162p3M184V mutant by intermittent prophylaxis with truvada. J Virol 2011;85(15):7933–6. http://dx.doi.org/10.1128/JVI.00843-11.

21. Parikh UM, Dobard C, Sharma S, et al. Complete protection from repeated vaginal simian-human immunodeficiency virus exposures in macaques by a topical gel containing tenofovir alone or with emtricitabine. J Virol 2009; 83(20):10358–65. http://dx.doi.org/10.1128/JVI.01073-09.

22. Garcia-Lerma JG, Heneine W. Animal models of antiretroviral prophylaxis for HIV prevention. Curr Opin HIV AIDS 2012;7(6):505–13. http://dx.doi.org/10.1097/COH.0b013e328358e484.

23. Abdool Karim Q, Abdool Karim SS, Frohlich JA, et al. Effectiveness and safety of tenofovir gel, an antiretroviral microbicide, for the prevention of HIV infection in women. Science 2010;329(5996):1168–74. http://dx.doi.org/10.1126/science.1193748.

24. Thigpen MC, Kebaabetswe PM, Paxton LA, et al. Antiretroviral preexposure prophylaxis for heterosexual HIV transmission in Botswana. N Engl J Med 2012; 367(5):423–34. http://dx.doi.org/10.1056/NEJMoa1110711.

25. Choopanya K, Martin M, Suntharasamai P, et al. Antiretroviral prophylaxis for HIV infection in injecting drug users in Bangkok, Thailand (The Bangkok Tenofovir Study): a randomised, double-blind, placebo-controlled phase 3 trial. Lancet 2013;381(9883):2083–90.

26. Grant RM, Lama JR, Anderson PL, et al. Preexposure chemoprophylaxis for HIV prevention in men who have sex with men. N Engl J Med 2010;363(27):2587–99. http://dx.doi.org/10.1056/NEJMoa1011205.

27. Baeten JM, Donnell D, Ndase P, et al. Antiretroviral prophylaxis for HIV prevention in heterosexual men and women. N Engl J Med 2012;367(5):399–410.

28. Van Damme L, Corneli A, Ahmed K, et al. Preexposure prophylaxis for HIV infection among African women. N Engl J Med 2012;367(5):411–22. http://dx.doi.org/10.1056/NEJMoa1202614.

29. McGowan I. An overview of antiretroviral pre-exposure prophylaxis of HIV infection. Am J Reprod Immunol 2014. http://dx.doi.org/10.1111/aji.12225.

30. Donnell D. Tenofovir disoproxil fumarate drug level indicate PrEP use is strongly correlated with HIV-1 protective effects: Kenya and Uganda [abstract 30]. In: Conference on Retroviruses and Opportunistic Infections. Seattle, March 5 - 8, 2012.

31. Martin M, Vanichseni S, Suntharasamai P, et al. Risk behaviors and risk factors for HIV infection among participants in the Bangkok Tenofovir study, an HIV preexposure prophylaxis trial among people who inject drugs. PLoS One 2014;9(3): e92809. http://dx.doi.org/10.1371/journal.pone.0092809.

32. Microbicide Trials Network. Microbicide trials network statement on decision to discontinue use of tenofovir gel in VOICE, a major HIV prevention study in women [media statement]. 2011. Available at: http://www.mtnstopshiv.org/node/3909. Accessed March 3, 2014.

33. Marrazzo J, Ramjee G, Nair G, et al. Pre-exposure prophylaxis for HIV in women: daily oral tenofovir, oral tenofovir/emtricitabine or vaginal tenofovir gel in the VOICE study (MTN 003) [abstract 26LB]. Conference on Retroviruses and Opportunistic Infections. Atlanta, March 3 - 6, 2013.

34. United States Food and Drug Administration (U.S. FDA). FDA approves first medication to reduce HIV risk [consumer update]. 2012. Available at: http://www.fda.gov/NewsEvents/Newsroom/PressAnnouncements/ucm312210.htm. Accessed March 28, 2014.

35. Centers for Disease Control and Prevention. Interim guidance: preexposure prophylaxis for the prevention of HIV infection in men who have sex with men. MMWR Morb Mortal Wkly Rep 2011;60(3):65–8.

36. Centers for Disease Control and Prevention. Interim guidance for clinicians considering the use of preexposure prophylaxis for the prevention of HIV infection in heterosexually active adults. MMWR Morb Mortal Wkly Rep 2012;61(31):586–9.

37. Centers for Disease Control and Prevention. Update to interim guidance for pre-exposure prophylaxis (PrEP) for the prevention of HIV infection: PrEP for injecting drug users. MMWR Morb Mortal Wkly Rep 2013;62(23):463–5.

38. Centers for Disease Control and Prevention. Preexposure Prophylaxis for the Prevention of HIV Infection in the United States, 2014. Clinical Practice Guideline. Available at http://www.cdc.gov/hiv/pdf/PrEPguidelines2014.pdf. Accessed September 16, 2014.

39. World Health Organization. Guidance on oral pre-exposure prophylaxis (PrEP) for serodiscordant couples, men and transgender women who have sex with men at high risk of HIV: recommendations for use in the context of demonstration projects. 2012. Available at: http://www.who.int/hiv/pub/guidance_prep/en/. Accessed April 12, 2014.

40. Gilead Sciences. Truvada for PrEP medication assistance program. Available at: http://www.gilead.com/responsibility/us-patient-access/truvada%20for%20prep%20medication%20assistance%20program. Accessed April 16, 2014.

41. HPTN 073, pre-exposure prophylaxis (PrEP) initiation and adherence among black men who have sex with men (BMSM) in three U.S. cities. Available at: http://www.hptn.org/research_studies/hptn073.asp. Accessed April 11, 2014.

42. AIDS Vaccine Advocacy Coalition. Achieving the end: one year and counting. 2013. Available at: http://www.avac.org/ht/d/sp/i/47457/pid/47457. Accessed April 11, 2014.

43. van de Vijver DA, Boucher CA. The risk of HIV drug resistance following implementation of pre-exposure prophylaxis. Curr Opin Infect Dis 2010;23(6):621–7.

44. Liegler T, Abdel-Mohsen M, Bentley LG, et al. HIV-1 drug resistance in the iPrEx pre-exposure prophylaxis trial. J Infect Dis 2014. [Epub ahead of print].

45. Ware NC, Wyatt MA, Haberer JE, et al. What's love got to do with it? Explaining adherence to oral antiretroviral pre-exposure prophylaxis for HIV-serodiscordant couples. J Acquir Immune Defic Syndr 2012;59(5):463–8.

46. Martin S, Elliott-DeSorbo DK, Calabrese S, et al. A comparison of adherence assessment methods utilized in the United States: perspectives of researchers, HIV-infected children, and their caregivers. AIDS Patient Care STDS 2009;23(8):593–601. http://dx.doi.org/10.1089/apc.2009.0021.

47. Muchomba FM, Gearing RE, Simoni JM, et al. State of the science of adherence in pre-exposure prophylaxis and microbicide trials. J Acquir Immune Defic Syndr 2012;61(4):490–8. http://dx.doi.org/10.1097/QAI.0b013e31826f9962.

48. Koenig LJ, Lyles C, Smith DK. Adherence to antiretroviral medications for HIV pre-exposure prophylaxis: lessons learned from trials and treatment studies. Am J Prev Med 2013;44(1 Suppl 2):S91–8. http://dx.doi.org/10.1016/j.amepre.2012.09.047.

49. Amico R, Liu A, McMahan V, et al. Adherence indicators and PrEP drug levels in the iPrEx study [abstract 92]. In: Conference on Retroviruses and Opportunistic Infections. Boston, February 27 - March 2, 2011.

50. Underhill K. Study designs for identifying risk compensation behavior among users of biomedical HIV prevention technologies: balancing methodological rigor and research ethics. Soc Sci Med 2013;94:115–23. http://dx.doi.org/10.1016/j.socscimed.2013.03.020.

51. Paxton LA. Considerations regarding antiretroviral chemoprophylaxis and heterosexuals in generalized epidemic settings. Curr Opin HIV AIDS 2012;7(6):557–62. http://dx.doi.org/10.1097/COH.0b013e328359064a.

52. Jiang J, Yang X, Ye L, et al. Pre-exposure prophylaxis for the prevention of HIV infection in high risk populations: a meta-analysis of randomized controlled trials. PLoS One 2014;9(2):e87674. http://dx.doi.org/10.1371/journal.pone.0087674.

53. Friend DR, Clark JT, Kiser PF, et al. Multipurpose prevention technologies: products in development. Antiviral Res 2013;100(Suppl):S39–47. http://dx.doi.org/10.1016/j.antiviral.2013.09.030.

54. Abraham BK, Gulick R. Next-generation oral preexposure prophylaxis: beyond tenofovir. Curr Opin HIV AIDS 2012;7(6):600–6. http://dx.doi.org/10.1097/COH.0b013e328358b9ce.

55. Andrews C, Gettie A, Russell-Lodrigue K, et al. Long-acting parenteral formulation of GSK1265744 protects macaques against repeated intrarectal challenges with SHIV [Abstract no. 24LB]; 20th Conference on Retroviruses and Opportunistic Infections; Atlanta, GA; March 3-6, 2013.

56. Andrews CD, Spreen WR, Mohri H, et al. Long-acting integrase inhibitor protects macaques from intrarectal simian/human immunodeficiency virus. Science 2014;343(6175):1151–4. http://dx.doi.org/10.1126/science.1248707.

57. Cohen J. Virology. A bid to thwart HIV with shot of long-lasting drug. Science 2014;343(6175):1067. http://dx.doi.org/10.1126/science.343.6175.1067.

58. van 't Klooster G, Hoeben E, Borghys H, et al. Pharmacokinetics and disposition of rilpivirine (TMC278) nanosuspension as a long-acting injectable antiretroviral formulation. Antimicrob Agents Chemother 2010;54(5):2042–50. http://dx.doi.org/10.1128/AAC.01529-09.

59. Lou M, Gould Y, Chen S, et al. Meta-analysis of safety data from 8 clinical studies with GSK1265744, an HIV integrase inhibitor, dosed orally or as injection of long-acting parenteral nanosuspension [abstract 1752] In: Interscience Conference on Antimicrobial Agents and Chemotherapy. Denver, September 10-13, 2013.

60. Margolis D, Bhatti B, Smith G, et al. Once-daily oral GSK1265744 (GSK744) as part of combination therapy in antiretroviral naïve adults: 24-week safety and efficacy results from the LATTE study [abstract LAI116482]. In: European AIDS Conference. Brussels, October 16-19, 2013.

61. Min S, DeJesus E, McCurdy L, et al. Pharmacokinetics (PK) and safety in healthy and HIV-infected subjects and short-term antiviral efficacy of S/GSK1265744, a next generation once daily HIV integrase inhibitor [abstract H-1228]. In: Interscience Conference on Antimicrobial Agents and Chemotherapy. San Francisco, September 12-15, 2009.

62. Spreen WR, Margolis DA, Pottage JC Jr. Long-acting injectable antiretrovirals for HIV treatment and prevention. Curr Opin HIV AIDS 2013;8(6):565–71. http://dx.doi.org/10.1097/COH.0000000000000002.

63. Spreen W, Min S, Ford SL, et al. Pharmacokinetics, safety, and monotherapy antiviral activity of GSK1265744, an HIV integrase strand transfer inhibitor. HIV Clin Trials 2013;14(5):192–203. http://dx.doi.org/10.1310/hct1405-192.

64. Spreen W, Ford S, Chen S, et al. Pharmacokinetics, safety and tolerability of the HIV integrase inhibitor S/GSK1265744 long acting parenteral nanosuspension following single dose administration to healthy adults [abstract TUPE040]. International AIDS Conference. Washington, DC, July 22-27, 2012.

65. Spreen W, Williams P, Margolis D, et al. First study of repeat dose co-administration of GSK1265744 and TMC278 long-acting parenteral nanosuspensions: pharmacokinetics, safety and tolerability in healthy adults. [abstract WEAB0103]. 7th International AIDS Society Conference on HIV Pathogenesis, Treatment and Prevention. Kuala Lumpur, June 30-July 3, 2013.

66. Pfizer. Maraviroc package insert. Available at: http://rsc.tech-res.com/safetyandpharmacovigilance/PIList.aspx. Accessed April 3, 2014.

67. Chan PL, Weatherley B, McFadyen L. A population pharmacokinetic meta-analysis of maraviroc in healthy volunteers and asymptomatic HIV-infected subjects. Br J Clin Pharmacol 2008;65(Suppl 1):76–85. http://dx.doi.org/10.1111/j.1365-2125.2008.03139.x.

68. HIV Prevention Trials Network. HPTN 069, Phase II randomized, double-blind, study of safety and tolerability of maraviroc, maraviroc + emtricitabine, maraviroc + tenofovir or tenofovir + emtricitabine for PreExposure prophylaxis to prevent HIV transmission in at-risk men who have sex with men and in at-risk women. Available at: http://www.hptn.org/research_studies/hptn069.asp. Accessed April 14, 2014.

69. Veazey RS, Springer MS, Marx PA, et al. Protection of macaques from vaginal SHIV challenge by an orally delivered CCR5 inhibitor. Nat Med 2005;11(12):1293–4.

70. Brown KC, Patterson KB, Malone SA, et al. Single and multiple dose pharmacokinetics of maraviroc in saliva, semen, and rectal tissue of healthy HIV-negative men. J Infect Dis 2011;203(10):1484–90. http://dx.doi.org/10.1093/infdis/jir059.

71. Fatkenheuer G, Pozniak AL, Johnson MA, et al. Efficacy of short-term monotherapy with maraviroc, a new CCR5 antagonist, in patients infected with HIV-1. Nat Med 2005;11(11):1170–2.

72. Dumond JB, Patterson KB, Pecha AL, et al. Maraviroc concentrates in the cervicovaginal fluid and vaginal tissue of HIV-negative women. J Acquir Immune Defic Syndr 2009;51(5):546–53. http://dx.doi.org/10.1097/QAI.0b013e3181ae69c5.

73. Neff CP, Ndolo T, Tandon A, et al. Oral pre-exposure prophylaxis by antiretrovirals raltegravir and maraviroc protects against HIV-1 vaginal transmission in a humanized mouse model. PLoS One 2010;5(12):e15257. http://dx.doi.org/10.1371/journal.pone.0015257.

74. Veazey RS, Ketas TJ, Dufour J, et al. Protection of rhesus macaques from vaginal infection by vaginally delivered maraviroc, an inhibitor of HIV-1 entry via the CCR5 co-receptor. J Infect Dis 2010;202(5):739–44. http://dx.doi.org/10.1086/655661.

75. Massud I. High maraviroc concentrations in rectal secretions after oral dosing do not prevent rectal SHIC transmissions in macaques. In: International AIDS Conference. Washington, DC, July 22-27, 2012.

76. Massud I, Aung W, Martin A, et al. Lack of prophylactic efficacy of oral mara-viroc in macaques despite high drug concentrations in rectal tissues. J Virol 2013;87(16):8952–61. http://dx.doi.org/10.1128/JVI.01204-13.

77. Fleishaker D, Wang X, Menon S, et al. A phase 2 study to assess the efficacy and safety of maraviroc, a CCR-5 antagonist in the treatment of rheumatoid arthritis. Arthritis Rheum 2009;60(Suppl 10):397.

78. Baert L, van 't Klooster G, Dries W, et al. Development of a long-acting inject-able formulation with nanoparticles of rilpivirine (TMC278) for HIV treatment. Eur J Pharm Biopharm 2009;72(3):502–8. http://dx.doi.org/10.1016/j.ejpb.2009.03.006.

79. Ford N, Lee J, Andrieux-Meyer I, et al. Safety, efficacy, and pharmacokinetics of rilpivirine: systematic review with an emphasis on resource-limited settings. HIV AIDS (Auckl) 2011;3:35–44. http://dx.doi.org/10.2147/HIV.S14559.

80. HIV Prevention Trials Network. HPTN studies in development. Available at: http://www.hptn.org/research_studies/Developing.asp. Accessed April 6, 2014.

81. Chen BA, Panther L, Hoesley C, et al. Safety and pharmacokinetics/pharmaco-dynamics of dapivirine and maraviroc vaginal rings [abstract #41]. Conference on Retroviruses and Opportunistic Infections 2014. March 3-6, 2014.

82. Rubtsova A, Wingood GM, Dunkle K, et al. Young adult women and correlates of potential adoption of pre-exposure prophylaxis (PrEP): results of a national sur-vey. Curr HIV Res 2013;11(7):543–8.

83. Yang D, Chariyalertsak C, Wongthanee A, et al. Acceptability of pre-exposure prophylaxis among men who have sex with men and transgender women in northern Thailand. PLoS One 2013;8(10):e76650. http://dx.doi.org/10.1371/journal.pone.0076650.

84. Underhill K, Morrow KM, Operario D, et al. Could FDA approval of pre-exposure prophylaxis make a difference? A qualitative study of PrEP acceptability and FDA perceptions among men who have sex with men. AIDS Behav 2014;18(2):241–9. http://dx.doi.org/10.1007/s10461-013-0498-9.

85. Galindo GR, Walker JJ, Hazelton P, et al. Community member perspectives from transgender women and men who have sex with men on pre-exposure prophy-laxis as an HIV prevention strategy: implications for implementation. Implement Sci 2012;7:116. http://dx.doi.org/10.1186/1748-5908-7-116.

86. Heffron R, Ngure K, Mugo N, et al. Willingness of Kenyan HIV-1 serodiscordant couples to use antiretroviral-based HIV-1 prevention strategies. J Acquir Im-mune Defic Syndr 2012;61(1):116–9. http://dx.doi.org/10.1097/QAI.0b013e31825da73f.

87. Krakower DS, Mimiaga MJ, Rosenberger JG, et al. Limited awareness and low immediate uptake of pre-exposure prophylaxis among men who have sex with men using an Internet social networking site. PLoS One 2012;7(3):e33119. http://dx.doi.org/10.1371/journal.pone.0033119.

88. Galea JT, Kinsler JJ, Salazar X, et al. Acceptability of pre-exposure prophylaxis as an HIV prevention strategy: barriers and facilitators to pre-exposure prophy-laxis uptake among at-risk Peruvian populations. Int J STD AIDS 2011;22(5):256–62. http://dx.doi.org/10.1258/ijsa.2009.009255.

89. HIV Prevention Trials Network. IPrExole. Available at: http://iprexole.com/1pages/community/spcommunity-links.php. Accessed March 9, 2014.

90. Cohen SE, Vittinghoff E, Anderson P, et al. Implementation of PrEP in STD clinics: high uptake and drug detection among MSM in the demonstration proj-ect [abstract 954]. In: Conference on Retroviruses and Opportunistic Infections. Boston, March 3-6, 2014.

91. Liu A, Cohen S, Follansbee S, et al. Early experiences implementing pre-exposure prophylaxis (PrEP) for HIV prevention in San Francisco. PLoS Med 2014;11(3):e1001613. http://dx.doi.org/10.1371/journal.pmed.1001613.

92. Cohen SE, Liu AY, Bernstein KT, et al. Preparing for HIV pre-exposure prophylaxis: lessons learned from post-exposure prophylaxis. Am J Prev Med 2013; 44(1 Suppl 2):S80–5. http://dx.doi.org/10.1016/j.amepre.2012.09.036.

93. National Association of State and Territorial AIDS Directors. Fact sheet: Pharmaceutical company patient assistance programs and Co-payment assistance programs for pre-exposure prophylaxis (PrEP) and post-exposure prophylaxis (PEP). Available at: https://start.truvada.com/Content/pdf/Medication_Assistance_Program.pdf. Accessed March 6, 2014.

94. Kirby T, Thornber-Dunwell M. Uptake of PrEP for HIV slow among MSM. Lancet 2014;383(9915):399–400.

95. Rawlings K, Mera R, Pechonkina A, et al. Status of truvada for HIV pre-exposure prophylaxis (PrEP) in the united states: an early drug utilization analysis [abstract H-663a]. In: Interscience Conference on Antimicrobial Agents and Chemotherapy. Denver, September 10-13, 2013.

96. Myers JE, Sepkowitz KA. A pill for HIV prevention: déjà vu all over again? Clin Infect Dis 2013;56(11):1604–12. http://dx.doi.org/10.1093/cid/cit085.

97. Marcus J, Buisker T, Horvath T, et al. Helping our patients take HIV pre-exposure prophylaxis (PrEP): a systematic review of adherence interventions. HIV Med 2014. http://dx.doi.org/10.1111/hiv.12132.

98. Amico KR, Mansoor LE, Corneli A, et al. Adherence support approaches in biomedical HIV prevention trials: experiences, insights and future directions from four multisite prevention trials. AIDS Behav 2013;17(6):2143–55. http://dx.doi.org/10.1007/s10461-013-0429-9.

99. Mills EJ, Nachega JB, Bangsberg DR, et al. Adherence to HAART: a systematic review of developed and developing nation patient-reported barriers and facilitators. PLoS Med 2006;3(11):e438.

100. Gupta RK, Van de Vijver DA, Manicklal S, et al. Evolving uses of oral reverse transcriptase inhibitors in the HIV-1 epidemic: from treatment to prevention. Retrovirology 2013;10:82. http://dx.doi.org/10.1186/1742-4690-10-82.

101. Horberg M, Raymond B. Financial policy issues for HIV pre-exposure prophylaxis: cost and access to insurance. Am J Prev Med 2013;44(1 Suppl 2): S125–8. http://dx.doi.org/10.1016/j.amepre.2012.09.039.

102. Karris MY, Beekmann SE, Mehta SR, et al. Are we prepped for preexposure prophylaxis (PrEP)? Provider opinions on the real-world use of PrEP in the United States and Canada. Clin Infect Dis 2014;58(5):704–12. http://dx.doi.org/10.1093/cid/cit796.

103. Krakower D, Mayer KH. Engaging healthcare providers to implement HIV pre-exposure prophylaxis. Curr Opin HIV AIDS 2012;7(6):593–9. http://dx.doi.org/10.1097/COH.0b013e3283590446.

104. Whiteside YO, Harris T, Scanlon C, et al. Self-perceived risk of HIV infection and attitudes about preexposure prophylaxis among sexually transmitted disease clinic attendees in South Carolina. AIDS Patient Care STDS 2011;25(6): 365–70. http://dx.doi.org/10.1089/apc.2010.0224.

105. Saberi P, Gamarel KE, Neilands TB, et al. Ambiguity, ambivalence, and apprehensions of taking HIV-1 pre-exposure prophylaxis among male couples in San Francisco: a mixed methods study. PLoS One 2012;7(11):e50061. http://dx.doi.org/10.1371/journal.pone.0050061.

106. White JM, Mimiaga MJ, Krakower DS, et al. Evolution of Massachusetts physician attitudes, knowledge, and experience regarding the use of antiretrovirals for HIV prevention. AIDS Patient Care STDS 2012;26(7):395–405. http://dx.doi.org/10.1089/apc.2012.0030.

107. Tripathi A, Ogbuanu C, Monger M, et al. Preexposure prophylaxis for HIV infection: Healthcare providers' knowledge, perception, and willingness to adopt future implementation in the southern US. South Med J 2012;105(4):199–206. http://dx.doi.org/10.1097/SMJ.0b013e31824f1a1b.

108. Arnold EA, Hazelton P, Lane T, et al. A qualitative study of provider thoughts on implementing pre-exposure prophylaxis (PrEP) in clinical settings to prevent HIV infection. PLoS One 2012;7(7):e40603. http://dx.doi.org/10.1371/journal.pone.0040603.

109. Mehta M, Semitala F, Lynen L, et al. Antiretroviral treatment in low-resource settings: what has changed in the last 10 years and what needs to change in the coming years? Expert Rev Anti Infect Ther 2012;10(11):1287–96. http://dx.doi.org/10.1586/eri.12.129.

110. Hellinger FJ. Assessing the cost effectiveness of pre-exposure prophylaxis for HIV prevention in the US. Pharmacoeconomics 2013;31(12):1091–104. http://dx.doi.org/10.1007/s40273-013-0111-0.

111. Alistar SS, Grant PM, Bendavid E. Comparative effectiveness and cost-effectiveness of antiretroviral therapy and pre-exposure prophylaxis for HIV prevention in South Africa. BMC Med 2014;12:46. http://dx.doi.org/10.1186/1741-7015-12-46.

112. Schackman BR, Eggman AA. Cost-effectiveness of pre-exposure prophylaxis for HIV: a review. Curr Opin HIV AIDS 2012;7(6):587–92. http://dx.doi.org/10.1097/COH.0b013e3283582c8b.

113. Hankins CA. Untangling the cost-effectiveness knot: who is oral antiretroviral HIV pre-exposure prophylaxis really for? Expert Rev Pharmacoecon Outcomes Res 2014;14(2):167–70. http://dx.doi.org/10.1586/14737167.2014.887447.

114. Juusola JL, Brandeau ML, Owens DK, et al. The cost-effectiveness of preexposure prophylaxis for HIV prevention in the United States in men who have sex with men. Ann Intern Med 2012;156(8):541–50. http://dx.doi.org/10.7326/0003-4819-156-8-201204170-00001.

115. Gostin LO, Kim SC. Ethical allocation of preexposure HIV prophylaxis. JAMA 2011;305(2):191–2. http://dx.doi.org/10.1001/jama.2010.1975.

116. Dutta MJ. Disseminating HIV pre-exposure prophylaxis information in underserved communities. Am J Prev Med 2013;44(1 Suppl 2):S133–6. http://dx.doi.org/10.1016/j.amepre.2012.09.030.

117. Baeten JM, Grant R. Use of antiretrovirals for HIV prevention: what do we know and what don't we know? Curr HIV/AIDS Rep 2013;10(2):142–51. http://dx.doi.org/10.1007/s11904-013-0157-9.

118. Project INFORM. Pre-exposure prophylaxis (PrEP). 2014. Available at: http://www.projectinform.org/prep/. Accessed April 1, 2014.

119. Massachusetts Department of Public Health. Frequently asked questions: pre-exposure prophylaxis (PrEP) for HIV infection Massachusetts Department of Public Health. 2013. Available at: http://www.mass.gov/eohhs/docs/dph/aids/prep-faq-providers.pdf. Accessed March 17, 2014.

120. Norton WE, Larson RS, Dearing JW. Primary care and public health partnerships for implementing pre-exposure prophylaxis. Am J Prev Med 2013;44(1 Suppl 2):S77–9. http://dx.doi.org/10.1016/j.amepre.2012.09.037.

121. De Man J, Colebunders R, Florence E, et al. What is the place of pre-exposure prophylaxis in HIV prevention? AIDS Rev 2013;15(2):102–11.

122. Aaron E, Cohan D. Preexposure prophylaxis for the prevention of HIV transmission to women. AIDS 2013;27(1):F1–5. http://dx.doi.org/10.1097/QAD.0b013e32835917b4.

123. Savasi V, Mandia L, Laoreti A, et al. Reproductive assistance in HIV serodiscordant couples. Hum Reprod Update 2013;19(2):136–50. http://dx.doi.org/10.1093/humupd/dms046.

124. Dearing JW, Smith DK, Larson RS, et al. Designing for Diffusion of a Biomedical Intervention. Am Journal of Preventive Medicine 2013;44(1):S70–6.

125. Smith DK, Beltrami J. A Proposed Framework to Monitor Daily Oral Antiretroviral Pre-Exposure Prophylaxis in the US. Am Journal of Preventive Medicine 2013;44(1):S141–6.

Barrier Methods for Human Immunodeficiency Virus Prevention

Ellen F. Eaton, MD*, Craig J. Hoesley, MD

KEYWORDS

- Human immunodeficiency virus prevention • Male condoms • Female condoms
- Microbicides

KEY POINTS

- Male condoms reduce human immunodeficiency virus transmission via homosexual and heterosexual intercourse by 80% to 90%.
- Male condoms are inexpensive, widely available, and easy to use, but nonadherence, improper use, and poor fit are the greatest barriers to consistent male condom usage.
- Female condoms are similar to male condoms in reducing sexually transmitted disease transmission, but their success has been limited by cost, study design, and delays in approval.
- Microbicides are a promising barrier to vaginal and rectal human immunodeficiency virus transmission.
- Only tenofovir-containing intravaginal gel has shown efficacy in preventing the sexual transmission of human immunodeficiency virus.

INTRODUCTION

For 3 decades, human immunodeficiency virus (HIV) has been a public health threat and priority, yet the incidence of new infections remains unchanged. Approximately 50,000 new HIV infections have occurred annually since the 1990s despite increased awareness, education, HIV screening, and the introduction of highly effective antiretrovirals.[1] Moreover, heterosexual transmission remains the most common cause of

Disclosure: The authors whose names are listed immediately above certify that they have no affiliations with or involvement in any organization or entity with any financial interest (such as honoraria; educational grants; participation in speakers' bureaus; membership, employment, consultancies, stock ownership, or other equity interest; and expert testimony or patent-licensing arrangements) or nonfinancial interest (such as personal or professional relationships, affiliations, knowledge or beliefs) in the subject matter or materials discussed in this article.
Division of Infectious Disease, University of Alabama, Birmingham, 229 Tinsley Harrison Tower, 1720 Second Avenue South, Birmingham, AL 35294, USA
* Corresponding author.
E-mail address: eeaton@uab.edu

Infect Dis Clin N Am 28 (2014) 585–599
http://dx.doi.org/10.1016/j.idc.2014.08.006
0891-5520/14/$ – see front matter © 2014 Elsevier Inc. All rights reserved.

id.theclinics.com

new infections worldwide.[2] Since early in the epidemic, condoms have been advocated as an effective physical barrier against HIV transmission. Studies have confirmed that latex condoms protect against HIV-sized particles and homosexual and heterosexual transmission of HIV.[3,4] Not only are condoms inexpensive and widely available, they are also safe, easy to use, and offer effective contraception and prevention against other sexually transmitted diseases.[5] Nonetheless, studies consistently show a 20% condom failure rate likely related to inappropriate or inconsistent usage. When used consistently and correctly, however, condoms reduce HIV infection by a factor of 10 to 20.[4]

Microbicides are a promising barrier to rectal and vaginal HIV transmission. Although several products with varying mechanisms of action have been studied, tenofovir and other antiretrovirals appear to be most effective at reducing viral transmission in animal and human studies.

MALE CONDOM
Types of Male Condoms

There are 3 main types of condoms: natural rubber latex condoms, synthetic condoms made from polyurethane and other latex-free materials, and membrane condoms made of lamb intestinal products. Latex condoms are well studied with regard to prevention of sexually transmitted infections (STIs) and HIV; synthetic condoms likely have similar effectiveness and are recommended for those with latex allergies. The membrane condom has not been found to reduce HIV transmission and is excluded from most studies of condom effectiveness.[3]

Indications

Condoms are recommended for heterosexual and homosexual intercourse and are protective for both partners. In addition to contraception, condoms offer a barrier against HIV and many STIs.[6] The risk of sexual transmission of HIV depends on several factors: sexual behavior, concurrent STIs, viral load of the infected partner, and circumcision.[7] The specific sexual act and the role of the infected partner also contribute to per-contact risk of HIV infection. For example, penile–anal intercourse poses a greater risk for HIV transmission than penile–vaginal intercourse.[4] The receptive role, whether anal or vaginal, also carries greatest risk.[4] A 2009 meta-analysis calculated a per-act risk of 0.04% in female-to-male transmission and 0.08% in male-to-female transmission in high-income countries.[7] The pooled estimate of infectivity per act of receptive anal intercourse was significantly higher at 1.7%. **Table 1** summarizes the per-act transmission risk of HIV based on sexual act according to

Table 1 The per-act transmission risk of HIV based on sexual act	
Transmission Mode	**Per-Act Risk of HIV Transmission**
Receptive anal intercourse	1.7%
High-income countries	
Female to male	0.04%
Male to female	0.08%
Low-income countries	
Female to male	0.38%
Male to female	0.38%

Boily and colleagues.[7] An African study of HIV-1 serodiscordant, heterosexual couples found a per-act transmission risk of 0.0019 and 0.0010, respectively, for unprotected male-to-female and female-to-male sexual transmission. This study also showed a 78% reduction in per-act risk of HIV infection with condom usage.[8] Condoms are also protective against herpes simplex virus, hepatitis B, Neisseria gonorrhea, Chlamydia trachomatis, and pelvic inflammatory disease.[9]

Effectiveness

Most research on HIV prevention studies serodiscordant couples with multiple exposures over time that are divided into 2 groups based on their behaviors: couples who always use condoms and those who never use condoms. By following up with HIV-negative partners over time and monitoring their serum for HIV antibodies, the rate of new HIV infections can be measured in partners who always use and those who never use condoms. Effectiveness is estimated by comparing incidence of HIV in each group with respect to their condom usage. Because most studies are observational and performed with imperfect use, they calculate effectiveness rather than efficacy, which requires perfect use. Couples are followed up with in observational studies, as it would be unethical to randomize some to condom usage and others to no condom use in a randomized, controlled trial based on condoms' proven protective properties. Lastly, couples should have no other risk factors for HIV infection like intravenous drug use or concomitant STIs, which would confound the study with new HIV infections independent of condom use.[2]

Most studies estimate that condoms reduce the per-contact risk of HIV transmission by 80% to 90%. By pooling seroconversion data in the early 1990s, one study estimated that consistent condom use reduced the per-contact rate of male-to-female HIV transmission by 94%.[4] A mathematical model of condom effectiveness derived from the same data showed that condoms decrease the per-contact probability of male-to-female transmission by a factor of 20.[4] A 2002 Cochrane review evaluated condoms in reducing HIV transmission in heterosexual serodiscordant couples and found them to be 82.9% effective.[2] This finding is consistent with that of the Partners in Prevention HSV/HIV Transmission Study, which studied African HIV-1 serodiscordant, heterosexual couples and found a 78% reduction in per-act risk of HIV infection with condom use.[8]

Research on condom effectiveness has been challenging, but incorporating new technology promises improved study design. For example, studies rely on individual reports of condom use, which is heavily influenced by participants' recall. Integration of mobile communication devices, such as cellular phones, has reduced recall bias by rapid behavior assessment and data collection. This technology allows daily reporting of sexual behavior thereby reducing bias. Specifically, one study found that 36.7% of participants reported unprotected vaginal sex via daily electronic reporting, but none reported unprotected vaginal sex when assessed via audio computer-assisted self-interviewing.[10] Mobile technology also holds promise for improved effectiveness via education and adherence. Many mobile device applications or "apps" are available for the prevention of HIV. One review found that most are infrequently downloaded and poorly rated by users.[11] Future research should focus on user-friendly mobile applications that educate and reinforce appropriate condom use.

Benefits

Condoms are widely available, discreet, inexpensive, and safe and provide contraception and STI prevention. Many clinics offer free condoms, but the estimated annual cost for couples who use them twice weekly is $150.[12] Condoms are also relatively easy to use. Finally, a recent study found that pleasure from penile-vaginal intercourse was not significantly different between those who did and those who did not use condoms.[13]

Limitations

Improper use, poor fit, and nonadherence are the greatest barriers to effective condom use. Condoms are known to slip and break, often from improper use rather than condom failure.[2] Condom errors are common: delayed application, applying with the wrong side out, improper lubrication, failure to leave space in receptacle tip, and premature removal. Furthermore, condom failure like breakage, slippage, poor fit and feel, and erection issues are well documented worldwide.[14] Self-reported breakage rates of 1% to 7% with anal and vaginal intercourse have been published.[9,15] One survey of women found that 36% reported an episode of condom breakage.[9] Condom slippage is less common, occurring 0.4% of the time.[15]

Appropriate use and condom integrity is essential for HIV prevention. A study by Warner and colleagues[16] evaluated the relationship between STIs and condom problems at an STI clinic. Of 336 participants, 41% reported that condoms broke, slipped, leaked or were not used throughout intercourse. Although no infections were found among those who denied user problems, 16.2% of those reporting condom user problems had incident chlamydia or gonorrhea.

Suboptimal condom fit and feel are directly related to condom errors and limit pleasure. Men reporting poor condom fit were 2.6 times more likely to experience condom breakage, 2.7 times more likely to experience condom slippage, and 2 times more likely to remove condoms prematurely during penile-vaginal sex.[10] Men reported poor fit led to less sexual pleasure for them and their female partners. An emphasis on improved design and education on proper use will likely improve condom use and reduce user and condom failure.

Adherence remains a barrier to consistent condom usage. Condom use requires consensual agreement between partners, and couples report that condoms interfere with pleasure and spontaneity.[17] In addition, alcohol use has been associated with unprotected sex.[17] Improving acceptability, accessibility, and affordability have allowed some communities to improve condom adherence. For example, Focus on the Future is an intervention for young, heterosexual African-American men that has successfully reduced the incidence of STIs, sexual partners, and unprotected sex. Focus on the Future provides an individual session with a trained peer who educates on correct condom use and emphasizes safe sex as a pleasurable experience without the infectious risk.[10] Jones and colleagues[18] used one initiative, called D-up, to reduce unprotected sex among young black men who have sex with men incorporating a popular opinion leader model. Participants were recruited, educated, and trained on communicating risk reduction techniques to their community. This model reduced unprotected anal intercourse in the community by 31.8% in 12 months. South Africa's national program improved condom adherence on a large scale by increasing condom popularity, integrating condom education into schools, and ensuring condom availability. Subsequently, condom use is increasing among youth and adults.[10]

FEMALE CONDOM

Female condoms became available in 1993 and were designed to give women control in intercourse and contraception. Because of gender and sexual inequality, many women are not able to negotiate male condom use with their partners, leading to unintended pregnancies and STI transmission. Female condoms may be inserted before intercourse, do not require consensual cooperation, and shield the introitus, vagina and cervix from direct penile contact and secretions. The timely introduction of the first female condom during the HIV epidemic provided an additional indication—HIV prevention during vaginal intercourse. The initial product struggled to gain acceptance and was cost prohibitive, but newer, more acceptable female condoms are promising options for safe sex. Nonetheless, the female condom remains an underutilized resource in the prevention of unintended pregnancy and STIs, specifically HIV.

Types of Female Condoms

Currently, multiple brands of female condoms are available, and most have a similar design: a sheath and internal and external retention features. The 17-cm sheath is made from polyurethane, synthetic latex or natural rubber latex. An insertion feature may be included and allows for product positioning. Female condoms are held in place with an external anchor, often a ring or frame, that limits invagination of the external portion into the vaginal canal and an internal retention feature such as a ring or sponge that prevents slippage outside of the vagina. In many products, the internal retention ring also serves as the insertion feature.[19]

The first female condom, the polyurethane Reality female condom, or FC1, was developed in the early 1990s. Although effective at contraception and STI transmission, the FC1 was expensive, costing almost 20 times more than the male condom.[20] Production of the FC1 ceased in 2009, and the few remaining products will expire in 2014. The second-generation female condom, FC2, is created from synthetic latex and has a slightly altered, seamless design. These changes allow mass production and reduce the cost of manufacturing.[19,20] As a result, FC2 production costs 25% less than FC1.[19] These improvements have increased availability in addition to affordability. The FC2 is prelubricated with silicon oil and, like many female condoms, is compatible with most lubricants. Both FC1 and FC2 have been approved for use by the World Health Organization (WHO) and the US Food and Drug Administration (FDA).

Cupid is the second female condom available globally for the public sector donor market and is approved for bulk procurement by the United Nations Population Fund. It includes a vanilla-scented latex sheath that is inserted with a sponge which also serves as an internal anchor. Cupid 2, a smaller product designed for Asian markets in which smaller male condoms are also used, is still undergoing testing and clinical trials.[19]

The Woman's Condom is a polyurethane sheath contained in a polyvinyl alcohol capsule (**Fig. 1**). After insertion, the capsule dissolves and releases the condom into position.[19] The condom is loosely anchored in place by several foam shapes lining the condom body. It is not prelubricated, but a water-based lubricant is provided. The Woman's condom is under review for approval by the WHO. The Phoenurse, Panty Condom, and Origami are all newer female condom options. The Panty Condom is unique in that a reusable panty serves as the external anchor.[19] **Table 2** summarizes the design and availability of several female condoms based on a review by Beksinska and colleagues[19] and the WHO.[20]

Indications

The female condom was designed for contraception and STI prevention and has been approved by the WHO for penile-vaginal intercourse. It has also been used for anal receptive sex by men and women.[21] Although this use is off label, future research will likely focus on the effectiveness of this practice.

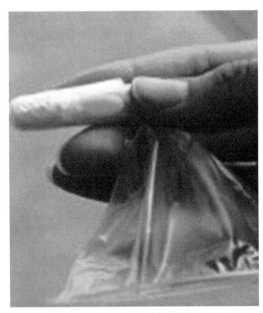

Fig. 1. The Woman's Condom. (*Photo courtesy* of PATH/Glenn Austin; with permission.)

Effectiveness

There are several challenges to consider when studying the effectiveness of female condoms in HIV prevention. Unlike male condoms, the structure of each female condom prototype varies as do the anticipated failure rates and performance. This challenges study design and testing and prolongs approval of new products. Also, the high cost of condom efficacy studies has led to more studies of functionality whereby surrogate measures such as condom breakage, slippage, and prostate-specific antigen levels in vaginal fluid are evaluated.[22,23] Functionality studies are quicker, easier, and less expensive but rely on the assumption that effective barriers to semen and pathogens translate to effective contraception and STI prevention.

In studying performance, female condoms were initially compared with male condoms, and more recently the FC1 has served as the reference standard. There are no direct head-to-head studies comparing male condoms with female condoms for HIV prevention. One study by French and colleagues[24] evaluated incident STIs among women provided with either male or female condoms. There was a nonsignificant reduction in STIs among those given female condoms, which suggests that female condoms are comparable in STI prevention. The first female condom, FC1, has the most research supporting its performance as contraception and STI prevention. A review of 137 articles and abstracts by Vijayakumar and colleagues[25] found that FC1 is effective at reducing STI incidence in women, but the authors report that data are limited and call for more research on performance rather than acceptability.

There are no data on FC2 effectiveness, but the FDA approved this product based on similarities to FC1 design and the results of a noninferiority trial comparing FC1 and FC2.[26] Studies have also found that FC2 has similar acceptability and breakage, slippage, and invagination rates when compared with FC1.[26,27]

The Woman's Condom, which has a novel dissolving insertion capsule, has comparable performance to the FC2 and low failure rates.[19] In addition, it was preferred over

Table 2
The design and availability of several female condoms based on a review by Beksinska and colleagues[19] and the WHO[20]

Model	Material	Insertion	Internal Retention	Outer Retention	UNFPA Approval
FC1	Polyurethane	Elastic ring	Elastic ring	Ring	Yes
FC2	Synthetic nitrile latex	Elastic ring	Elastic ring	Ring	Yes
Woman's Condom	Polyurethane	Dissolving capsule	Foam pads	Ring	Under review
Cupid 1	Natural rubber	Sponge	Sponge	Semirigid frame	Yes
Phoenurse	Polyurethane	Elastic ring	Elastic ring	Ring	Under review
Panty Condom	Synthetic polyethylene resin	Finger or penis	NA	Panty	Under review
Origami	Silicone	TBD	NA	Circular phalange	Not yet applied
VA w.o.w.	Natural rubber	Sponge	Sponge	Semirigid frame	Under review

Abbreviations: NA, not applicable; TBD, to be determined.

the FC2 and VA w.o.w. for appearance, ease of use, and fit in a randomized, crossover study of women in South Africa.[28] A randomized, controlled, noninferiority trial in China and South Africa evaluated FC2, VA w.o.w., Woman's Condom, and the Cupid 1 condom. Noninferiority for failure events was observed for all 3 models when compared with FC2.[29]

Benefits

The female condom affords women control over contraception and safe sex practices. It does not require a prescription or a health care provider, has no significant side effects, and is safely used with many oil- and water-based lubricants. It does not interfere with female hormones, allowing a reversible contraception, and the external ring may enhance pleasure during intercourse. Female condom availability is on the increase—the distribution of female condoms doubled from 2007 to 2010.[19]

Limitations

Use of the female condom is limited largely because of acceptability and cost.[30] A prospective study of women deemed high risk for STIs found that one-third of women provided with FC1 used it no more than twice, and another 15% did not use them at all.[31] Although new female condoms have a more economical design, they still cost significantly more than the male condom. A 2012 estimate for the FC2 was US $0.57 per unit.[19] Female condoms are less readily available at convenience stores, supermarkets, and drug stores than male condoms. Female condoms represent 0.19% of worldwide condom purchases.[19] This fact likely reflects limited demand and supply. Costly and labor-intensive regulatory processes have delayed development and approval of newer products. As a result, promising new models, such as the Origami and Panty Condom, have not received approval for mass distribution.

Like male condoms, female condom effectiveness is limited by user problems and may be even less user friendly than male condoms. One Brazilian study found that women reported more user problems and higher failure rates with female condoms than the male condom despite education on proper use.[22] Female condoms may slip in or out of the vagina and break or tear. In addition, there is a chance for penile exposure with misdirection when the penis is inserted into the vagina but outside of the female condom sheath.

Future Directions

Male and Female condom producers are now focusing on making condoms more attractive by adding features aimed at enhancing sexual pleasure. The condom industry and public health advocates appreciate that the condom's greatest limitation is acceptability. The Bill and Melinda Gates Foundation is one such global health advocate that has offered grants for the development of pleasure-enhancing condoms.[32] **Table 3** is a summary of novel male condoms with features promising rapid application and sexual pleasure.[32,33]

MICROBICIDES

Microbicides are a promising HIV prevention strategy. They are self-administered compounds that can be applied topically in the vagina or rectum in effort to prevent or significantly reduce the acquisition of HIV (and possibly other sexually transmitted pathogens) during sexual activity. Microbicides could potentially be delivered in multiple formulations, including gels, creams, films, sponges, or intravaginal rings. More than 50 candidate topical microbicide compounds have undergone preclinical or

Table 3
Summary of novel male condoms with features promising rapid application and sexual pleasure

Product	Features
InSpiral	Spiral-shaped material intended to stimulate
eZ-On	Can be put on in either direction
Durex Play-Ring of Bliss	Vibrating condom ring
4:Secs	Ring-shaped applicator splits apart for rapid application
Origami	Loose pleats allow movement designed to stimulate
Cambridge Design Partnership prototype	Material will tighten during intercourse
Kimbranox Ltd prototype	Rapidom applicator allows rapid, fool-proof application

clinical testing in the last 10 years, but there are currently no FDA-approved compounds. To date, only tenofovir-containing intravaginal gel has shown efficacy in preventing the sexual transmission of HIV.

Mechanisms of Action

The mechanism of action of the candidate microbicides studied thus far can be broadly classified into 5 categories: (1) surfactants, which inactivate surface pathogens by disrupting membranes; (2) buffering agents, which maintain or enhance natural defenses in the vagina; (3) blocking agents, which develop a barrier between potential pathogens and receptive mucosal host cells; (4) inhibition of HIV fusion via coreceptor blockade; and (5) HIV replication inhibition in infected host cells. **Table 4** outlines the categories of microbicide compounds and specific examples.

Safety and Effectiveness

Surfactants
Surfactants or detergents are agents capable of destroying the integrity of cell membranes, including viral envelopes, by solubilizing lipids or denaturing proteins. Nonoxynol-9 (N-9) is a surfactant that was originally developed in the 1960s as a spermicide and was the first compound evaluated as a vaginal microbicide. Despite efficacy in animal models, an N-9–containing vaginal gel failed to prevent HIV transmission in a randomized, placebo-controlled clinical trial in commercial sex workers.[34,35] Moreover, the HIV transmission rate was somewhat higher in the N-9 group compared with those women who received the placebo gel, suggesting N-9 had an abrasive impact on mucosal tissue, which could enhance transmission.[36]

Table 4
Mechanism of action of candidate microbicides

Action	Candidate Microbicide Examples
Surfactants	Nonoxynol-9 (N-9), C31G (SAVVY), sodium lauryl sulfate (Invisible Condom)
Buffers	BufferGel, lactobacillus suppositories
Blockers	Carraguard, cellulose sulfate, PRO2000
HIV fusion inhibitors	Maraviroc, PSC-RANTES, C34
HIV replication inhibitors	Tenofovir, dapivirine, UC781, MIV150

C31G (SAVVY) is a surfactant with in vitro activity against HIV, herpes simplex virus, and some bacteria, including Chlamydia trachomatis.[37] However, in placebo-controlled clinical trials performed in Ghana and Nigeria, C31G vaginal gel did not prevent HIV transmission.[38,39] Like N-9, C31G gel was associated with significant reproductive tract adverse events, suggesting safety concerns. Sodium lauryl sulfate (Invisible Condom) is another surfactant formulated as a vaginal gel for the prevention of HIV infection. In a phase 2 clinic trial in Cameroon, this compound was found to be safe and acceptable but has not yet undergone assessment for HIV prevention effectiveness.[40] To date, the clinical trial results for surfactants as vaginal microbicides have been disappointing, suggesting a viable microbicide candidate will not be derived from this class of agents.

Buffers

The pH of cervicovaginal fluid is acidic (3.5–4.5) which contributes to innate immunity against sexually transmitted pathogens, including HIV. An elevation in vaginal pH can occur with the presence of semen (pH level, 7.0–8.0) or a reduction of lactobacilli. Lactobacilli are vaginal flora bacteria that produce hydrogen peroxide and lactic acid, thus, contributing to the natural acidic environment of the vagina. Compounds, including the provision of exogenous lactobacilli via suppositories, which can preserve the acidic pH of the vaginal milieu, could theoretically protect against HIV infection and other STIs.[41] BufferGel, a polyacrylic acid, is capable of buffering twice its volume in semen to a pH level of 5 or less and has in vitro activity against HIV, herpes simplex virus, and human papilloma virus. However, BufferGel was not able to prevent HIV infection in a large clinical trial.[42] Early research into other candidates that maintain or enhance vaginal defenses includes Acidform, a buffering agent, and the use of live recombinant Lactobacillus species.[43,44]

Blockers

Anionic or sulfonated polymers have the capacity to inhibit HIV adsorption and fusion with a receptive host cell. PRO2000 vaginal gel is a sulfonated polymer with in vitro activity against HIV, herpes simplex virus, C trachomatis, and Neisseria gonorrhoeae.[45] However, it was proven ineffective in preventing HIV infection in women in a clinical trial.[42] Carraguard, a sulfated polysaccharide compound derived from red seaweed, blocks HIV infection of cervical epithelial cells and prevents trafficking of HIV-infected macrophages to lymph nodes.[46] It did not result in reduction of HIV acquisition during sexual activity when compared with placebo in South African women.[47] Cellulose sulfate, a polyanion, has also been formulated as a vaginal gel and, despite in vitro anti-HIV and spermicidal properties, was ineffective in preventing HIV infection in a phase 3 clinical trial.[48,49] This class of candidate microbicides is no longer considered a viable option for microbicide development.

Human immunodeficiency virus fusion inhibitors

A critical step in the HIV lifecycle is the binding of HIV to specific chemokine receptors (ie, CCR5 and CXCR4) on the cell surface. Molecules capable of attaching to these HIV coreceptors on the surface of receptive host cells in the anogenital tract could potentially be effective candidate microbicides. Maraviroc, a small molecule drug, binds to the CCR5 receptor and is FDA-approved for the treatment of HIV infection. It has been formulated as a gel and impregnated in a vaginal ring for assessment as a microbicide.[50] PSC-RANTES is a recombinant chemokine analogue that functions as a CCR5 inhibitor. It has been shown to provide protection against vaginal challenge of simian immunodeficiency virus infection in rhesus macaques, but its development as a microbicide in humans may be limited by production costs as a recombinant agent.[51] Several other HIV-specific fusion and entry inhibitors are in the microbicide preclinical development pipeline line, but, to date, none of the agents in this class have been assessed for HIV prevention effectiveness in phase 3 clinical trials.

Human immunodeficiency virus replication inhibitors

The microbicide development pathway is currently dominated by antiretroviral compounds. Tenofovir is a nucleotide analogue that inhibits reverse transcriptase and is an FDA-approved drug for the treatment of HIV infection. It was formulated as a vaginal gel and was the first antiretroviral agent utilized as microbicide. In the CAPRISA (center for the AIDS program of research in South Africa) 004 clinical trial, intravaginal administration of tenofovir gel before and after sexual intercourse resulted in an overall 39% reduction in HIV incidence. In women with consistent use of the gel, the HIV incidence was reduced even further (54%).[52] This clinical trial has provided the first and only data proving a microbicide can be an effective HIV prevention tool. The VOICE (vaginal and oral interventions to control the epidemic) trial examined the safety and effectiveness of intravaginal tenofovir gel and 2 oral antiretroviral agents (Viread [tenofovir disoproxil fumarate] and Truvada [tenofovir disoproxil fumarate-emtricitabine]) taken daily to reduce the risk of HIV acquisition in women. Interim results showed oral and intravaginal tenofovir failed to show any effective decrease in HIV transmission. The HIV incidence was similar in women using the tenofovir and placebo intravaginal gels.[53] The reasons for the conflicting results of the CAPRISA 004 and VOICE trials have not been fully elucidated, but participant adherence is a likely contributing factor.[54] The ongoing FACTS (follow-on African Consortium for tenofovir studies) 001 clinical trial is also testing the effectiveness of coitally-dependent tenofovir intravaginal gel and will hopefully confirm the findings of the CAPRISA 004 trial.

Dapivirine, a nonnucleoside reverse transcriptase inhibitor, has been formulated as a vaginal gel and as a vaginal ring. Both formulations are found to be safe and acceptable, and an ongoing phase 3 clinical trial of the dapivirine vaginal ring will provide effectiveness data in the near future.[55,56] Another nonnucleoside reverse transcriptase inhibitor, UC781, has shown promise as a microbicide candidate, but development has been limited secondary to the drug's poor water solubility and difficulty in identifying a viable delivery method.[57]

Antiretroviral drugs are also being evaluated in combination with other compounds in an effort to enhance the activity of microbicides. For example, MIV150, a nonnucleoside reverse transcriptase inhibitor, has been combined with carrageenan and zinc acetate in a vaginal gel. This combination microbicide has shown efficacy in preventing simian immunodeficiency virus transmission, human papillomavirus, and herpes simplex virus in animal models.[58,59] Future microbicide compounds are being considered, which would combine anti-HIV agents with contraceptives.

Rectal Microbicides

Unprotected receptive anal intercourse among HIV serodiscordant couples is recognized as an efficient method for viral transmission. This sexual practice is common among men who have sex with men (MSM) and is likely an underestimated heterosexual activity as well.[60,61] The risk of HIV acquisition associated with heterosexual unprotected receptive anal intercourse is 1.7%, whereas it is only 0.08% during unprotected vaginal intercourse.[7] These data emphasize the need to develop novel prevention strategies in populations at risk of acquiring HIV infection through receptive anal intercourse who are not willing to utilize condoms. Recent phase 1 rectal microbicides have studied the safety, acceptability, and pharmacokinetics of 2 separate gels containing UC781 and tenofovir.[62,63] In both studies, the gel was deemed safe and highly acceptable. The tenofovir gel formulation used in vaginal studies was not well tolerated when inserted into the rectum, which resulted in the development of a reduced glycerin formulation for rectal studies. Currently, there is an ongoing phase 2 study of the rectally applied tenofovir with reduced glycerin gel.

REFERENCES

1. Hall HI, Song R, Rhodes P, et al. Estimation of HIV incidence in the United States. JAMA 2008;300(5):520–9.
2. Weller S, Davis K. Condom effectiveness in reducing heterosexual HIV transmission [review]. Cochrane Database Syst Rev 2002;(1):CD003255.
3. Carey RF, Lytle CD, Cyr WH. Implications of laboratory tests of condom integrity. Sex Transm Dis 1999;26(4):216–20.
4. Pinkerton SD, Abramson PR. Effectiveness of condoms in preventing HIV transmission. Soc Sci Med 1997;44(9):1303–12.
5. Holmes KK. Effectiveness of condoms in preventing sexually transmitted infections. Bull World Health Organ 2004;82:454–61.
6. Centers for Disease Control and Prevention. Update: barrier protection against HIV and other sexually transmitted diseases. MMWR Morb Mortal Wkly Rep 1993;42:589–91.
7. Boily MC, Baggaley RF, Wang L, et al. Heterosexual risk of HIV-1 infection per sexual act: systematic review and meta-analysis of observational studies [review]. Lancet Infect Dis 2009;9(2):118–29. http://dx.doi.org/10.1016/S1473-3099(09)70021-0.
8. Hughes JP, Baeten JM, Lingappa JR, Partners in Prevention HSV/HIV Transmission Study Team. Determinants of per-coital-act HIV-1 infectivity among African HIV-1-serodiscordant couples. J Infect Dis 2012;205(3):358.
9. Cates W, Stone KM. Family planning, sexually transmitted diseases, and contraceptive choice: a literature update. Fam Plann Perspect 1992;24:75–84.
10. Crosby RA. State of condom use in HIV prevention science and practice [review]. Curr HIV/AIDS Rep 2013;10(1):59–64. http://dx.doi.org/10.1007/s11904-012-0143-7.
11. Muessig KE, Pike EC, Legrand S, et al. Mobile phone applications for the care and prevention of HIV and other sexually transmitted diseases: a review [review]. J Med Internet Res 2013;15(1):e1. http://dx.doi.org/10.2196/jmir.2301.
12. Palmer K. The real cost of birth control. US News World Rep. 2010. Available at: http://money.usnews.com/money/blogs/alpha-consumer/2010/08/27/the-real-cost-of-birth-control. Accessed February 5, 2014.
13. Sanders SA, Reece M, Herbenick D, et al. Condom use during most recent vaginal intercourse event among a probability sample of adults in the United States. J Sex Med 2010;7(Suppl 5):362–73. http://dx.doi.org/10.1111/j.1743-6109.2010.02011.x.
14. Sanders SA, Yarber WL, Kaufman EL, et al. Condom use errors and problems: a global view [review]. Sex Health 2012;9(1):81–95. http://dx.doi.org/10.1071/SH11095.
15. Trussell JE, Warner DL, Hatcher R. Condom performance during vaginal intercourse: comparison of Trojan-Enz (trademark) and Tactylon (trademark) condoms. Contraception 1992;45:11–9.
16. Warner L, Newman DR, Kamb ML, et al, Project RESPECT Study Group. Problems with condom use among patients attending sexually transmitted disease clinics: prevalence, predictors, and relation to incident gonorrhea and chlamydia. Am J Epidemiol 2008;167(3):341–9.

17. Curran K, Baeten JM, Coates TJ, et al. HIV-1 prevention for HIV-1 serodiscordant couples. Curr HIV/AIDS Rep 2012;9(2):160–70.

18. Jones KT, Gray P, Whiteside YO, et al. Evaluation of an HIV prevention intervention adapted for black men who have sex with men. Am J Public Health 2008; 98(6):1043–50. http://dx.doi.org/10.2105/AJPH.2007.120337.

19. Beksinska M, Smit J, Joanis C, et al. New female condoms in the pipeline. Reprod Health Matters 2012;20(40):188–96. http://dx.doi.org/10.1016/S0968-8080(12)40659-0.

20. The WHO/UNFPA Female Condom Technical Review Committee. Department of reproductive health and research. Report on FC2. Available at: http://whqlibdoc.who.int/hq/2007/WHO_RHR_07.18_eng.pdf?ua=1. Accessed January 25, 2014.

21. Kelvin EA, Mantell JE, Candelario N, et al. Off-label use of the female condom for anal intercourse among men in New York City. Am J Public Health 2011; 101(12):2241–4. http://dx.doi.org/10.2105/AJPH.2011.300260.

22. Galvão LW, Oliveira LC, Díaz J, et al. Effectiveness of female and male condoms in preventing exposure to semen during vaginal intercourse: a randomized trial. Contraception 2005;71(2):130.

23. Macaluso M, Blackwell R, Jamieson DJ, et al. Efficacy of the male latex condom and of the female polyurethane condom as barriers to semen during intercourse: a randomized clinical trial. Am J Epidemiol 2007;166(1):88–96.

24. French PP, Latka M, Gollub EL, et al. Use-effectiveness of the female versus male condom in preventing sexually transmitted disease in women. Sex Transm Dis 2003;30(5):433–9.

25. Vijayakumar G, Mabude Z, Smit J, et al. A review of female-condom effectiveness: patterns of use and impact on protected sex acts and STI incidence [review]. Int J STD AIDS 2006;17(10):652–9.

26. Beksinska M, Smit J, Mabude Z, et al. Performance of the reality polyurethane female condom and a synthetic latex prototype: a randomized crossover trial among South African women. Contraception 2006;73(4):386–93.

27. Smit J, Beksinska M, Vijayakumar G, et al. Short-term acceptability of the Reality polyurethane female condom and a synthetic latex prototype: a randomized crossover trial among South African women. Contraception 2006;73(4):394.

28. Joanis C, Beksinska M, Hart C, et al. Three new female condoms: which do South-African women prefer? Contraception 2011;83(3):248–54. http://dx.doi.org/10.1016/j.contraception.2010.08.002.

29. Beksinska M, Piaggio G, Smit JA, et al. Performance and safety of the second-generation female condom (FC2) versus the Woman's, the VA worn-of-women, and the Cupid female condoms: a randomised controlled non-inferiority crossover trial. Lancet Glob Health 2013;1:e146–52.

30. Laga M, Piot P. Prevention of sexual transmission of HIV: real results, science progressing, societies remaining behind [review]. AIDS 2012;26(10):1223–9. http://dx.doi.org/10.1097/QAD.0b013e32835462b8.

31. Macaluso M, Demand M, Artz L, et al. Female condom use among women at high risk of sexually transmitted disease. Fam Plann Perspect 2000;32(3): 138–44.

32. Belluck P. Getting men to want to use condoms. NYT.com. 2013. Available at: http://well.blogs.nytimes.com. Accessed February 22, 2014.

33. Bill and Melinda Gates Foundation. Gates Foundation awards grants to test ideas ranging from using big data for social good to inventing the next generation of condoms. Grandchallenges.org. 2013. Available at: http://www.grandchallenges.org/. Accessed February 22, 2014.

34. Miller CJ, Alexander NJ, Gettie A, et al. The effect of contraceptives containing nonoxynol-9 on the genital transmission of simian immunodeficiency virus in rhesus macaques. Fertil Steril 1992;57(5):1126–8.

35. Van Damme L, Ramjee G, Alary M, et al. Effectiveness of COL-1492, a nonoxynol-9 vaginal gel, on HIV-1 transmission in female sex workers: a randomized controlled trial. Lancet 2002;360(9338):971–7.

36. Stafford MK, Ward H, Flanagan A, et al. Safety study of nonoxynol-9 as a vaginal microbicide: evidence of adverse effects. J Acquir Immune Defic Syndr Hum Retrovirol 1998;17(4):327–31.

37. Wyrick PB, Knight ST, Gerbig DG, et al. The microbicidal agent C31G inhibits Chlamydia trachomatis infectivity in vitro. Antimicrob Agents Chemother 1997; 41(6):1335–44.

38. Peterson L, Nanada K, Opoku BK, et al. SAVVY (C31G) gel for prevention of HIV infection in women: a phase 3, double blind, randomized, placebo-controlled trial in Ghana. PLoS One 2007;2(12):e1312.

39. Feldblum PJ, Adeiga A, Bakare R, et al. SAVVY vaginal gel (C31G) for prevention of HIV infection: a randomized controlled trial in Nigeria. PLoS One 2008; 3(1):e1474.

40. Mbopi-Keou FX, Trottier S, Omar RF, et al. A randomized, double-blind, placebo-controlled phase II extended safety study of two invisible condom formulations in Cameroonian women. Contraception 2010;81(1):79–85.

41. Martin HL, Richardson BA, Nyange PM, et al. Vaginal lactobacilli, microbial flora, and risk of human immunodeficiency virus type 1 and sexually transmitted disease acquisition. J Infect Dis 1999;180(6):1863–8.

42. Abdool Karim SS, Richardson BA, Ramjee G, et al. Safety and effectiveness of buffergel and 0.5% PRO2000 gel for the prevention of HIV infection in women. AIDS 2011;25(7):957–66.

43. Amaral E, Faundes A, Zaneveld L, et al. Study of the vaginal tolerance to acidiform, an acid-buffering, bioadhesive gel. Contraception 1999;60(6):361–6.

44. Lagenaur LA, Sanders-Beer BE, Brichacek B, et al. Prevention of vaginal SHIV transmission in macaques by a live recombinant Lactobacillus. Nature 2011;4: 648–57.

45. Keller MJ, Zerhouni-Layachi B, Chesshenko N, et al. PRO2000 gel inhibits HIV and herpes simplex virus infection following vaginal application: a double-blind placebo-controlled trial. J Infect Dis 2006;193(1):27–35.

46. Perotti ME, Pirovano A, Phillips DM. Carageenan formulation prevents macrophage trafficking from vagina: implications for microbicide development. Biol Reprod 2003;69(3):933–9.

47. Skoler-Karpoff S, Ramjee G, Ahmed K, et al. Efficacy of carraguard for prevention of HIV infection in women in South Africa: a randomized, double-blind, placebo-controlled trial. Lancet 2008;372(9654):1977–87.

48. Scordi-Bello IA, Mosoian A, He C, et al. Candidate sulfonated and sulfated topical microbicides: comparison of anti-human immunodeficiency virus activities and mechanisms of action. Antimicrob Agents Chemother 2005;49(9): 3607–15.

49. Halpern V, Ogunsola F, Obunge O, et al. Effectiveness of cellulose sulfate vaginal gel for the prevention of HIV infection: results of a phase III trial in Nigeria. PLoS One 2008;3(11):e3784.

50. Veazey RS, Ketas TJ, Dufour J, et al. Protection of rhesus macaques from vaginal infection by vaginally delivered maraviroc, an inhibitor of HIV-1 entry via the CCR5 co-receptor. J Infect Dis 2010;202(5):739–44.

51. Veazey RS, Ling B, Green LC, et al. Topically applied recombinant chemokine analogues fully protect macaques from vaginal simian immunodeficiency virus challenge. J Infect Dis 2009;199(10):1525–7.
52. Abdool Karim Q, Abdool Karim SS, Frohlich JA, et al. Effectiveness and safety of tenofovir gel, an antiretroviral microbicide, for the prevention of HIV infection in women. Science 2010;329:1168–74.
53. Microbicide Trials Network. MTN statement on decision to discontinue use of tenofovir gel in VOICE, a major HIV prevention study in women. 2011. Available at: http://clinicaltrials.gov/ct2/show/NCT00705679. Accessed February 5, 2014.
54. Van der Straten A, Van Damme L, Haberer JE, et al. Unraveling the divergent results of pre-exposure prophylaxis trials for HIV prevention. AIDS 2012;26(7): F13–9.
55. Nel AM, Coplan P, van de Wijgert JH, et al. Safety, tolerability, and systemic absorption of dapivirine vaginal microbicide gel in healthy, HIV-negative women. AIDS 2009;23(12):1531–8.
56. Romano J, Variano B, Coplan P, et al. Safety and availability of dapivirine (TMC120) delivered from an intravaginal ring. AIDS Res Hum Retroviruses 2009;25:483–8.
57. Van Herrewege Y, Michiels J, Van Roey J, et al. In vitro evaluation of nonnucleoside reverse transcriptase inhibitors UC-781 and TMC120-R147681 as human immunodeficiency virus microbicides. Antimicrob Agents Chemother 2004;48(1): 337–9.
58. Singer R, Derby N, Rodriguez A, et al. The nonnucleoside reverse transcriptase inhibitor MIV-150 in carageenan gel prevents rectal transmission of simian/human immunodeficiency virus infection in macaques. J Virol 2011;85(11): 5504–12.
59. Fernandez-Romero JA, Abraham CJ, Rodriguez A, et al. Zinc acetate/carrageenan gels exhibit potent activity in vivo against high-dose herpes simplex virus 2 vaginal and rectal challenge. Antimicrob Agents Chemother 2012; 56(1):358–68.
60. Wolitski RJ, Fenton KA. Sexual health, HIV, and sexually transmitted infections among gay, bisexual, and other men who have sex with men in the United States. AIDS Behav 2011;15(S1):S9–17.
61. Gorbach PM, Manhart LE, Hess KL, et al. Anal intercourse among heterosexuals in three sexually transmitted disease clinics in the Unites States. Sex Transm Dis 2009;36(4):193–8.
62. Anton PA, Saunders T, Elliott J, et al. First phase 1 double-blind, placebo-controlled, randomized rectal microbicide trial using UC781 gel with a novel index of ex vivo efficacy. PLoS One 2011;6(9):e23243.
63. McGowan I, Hoesley C, Cranston RD, et al. A phase 1 randomized, double blind, placebo controlled rectal safety and acceptability study of tenofovir 1% gel (MTN-007). PLoS One 2013;8(4):e60147.

Prevention of Human Immunodeficiency Virus and AIDS

Postexposure Prophylaxis (Including Health Care Workers)

Susan E. Beekmann, RN, MPH[a], David K. Henderson, MD[b],*

KEYWORDS

- HIV • Postexposure prophylaxis • Occupational exposure
- Nonoccupational exposure • HIV PEP

KEY POINTS

- HIV PEP is intended to prevent HIV infection after an exposure.
- HIV PEP is one of several strategies for HIV prevention.
- PEP was first used after occupational HIV exposures.
- A case-control study of HIV seroconversion in health care workers after percutaneous exposure published in 1997 provided the first evidence in humans that PEP with a single antiretroviral agent seemed to be protective against infection.
- Use of PEP has been extended to nonoccupational exposures, including following sexual contact or injection-drug use.

Although human immunodeficiency virus (HIV) incidence in the United States was relatively stable from 2006 to 2009, a total of 48,100 new HIV infections were estimated to have occurred in 2009 in the United States[1] and 2.3 million new cases occurred globally in 2012.[2] Postexposure prophylaxis (PEP), which is designed to prevent HIV infection after an exposure, is one of several strategies for HIV prevention. PEP was first used after occupational HIV exposures in the late 1980s, with the Centers for Disease Control and Prevention (CDC) issuing the first set of guidelines that included considerations regarding the use of antiretroviral agents for PEP after occupational HIV exposures in

Disclosure Statement: The authors have nothing to disclose.
[a] Department of Internal Medicine, The University of Iowa College of Medicine, Infectious Diseases SW34-J GH, Iowa City, IA 52242, USA; [b] Clinical Center, National Institutes of Health, Bethesda, Building 10-CRC, Rm 6-2551, MD 20892, USA
* Corresponding author.
E-mail address: DHenderson@cc.nih.gov

Infect Dis Clin N Am 28 (2014) 601–613
http://dx.doi.org/10.1016/j.idc.2014.08.005
0891-5520/14/$ – see front matter © 2014 Elsevier Inc. All rights reserved.

1990.[3] A case-control study of HIV seroconversion in health care workers (HCW) after percutaneous exposure published in 1997 provided the first evidence in humans that PEP with a single antiretroviral agent seemed to be protective against infection.[4] More recently, use of PEP has been extended to nonoccupational exposures, including after sexual contact or injection-drug use.[5] This article provides a brief rationale for PEP, assessment of the need for PEP, and details of its implementation.

RATIONALE FOR POSTEXPOSURE PROPHYLAXIS FOR EXPOSURES TO HUMAN IMMUNODEFICIENCY VIRUS
Biologic Plausibility of Postexposure Prophylaxis

The hypothesis underlying the administration of antiretroviral chemoprophylaxis is that postexposure treatment provided during a "window of opportunity" will attenuate initial HIV replication and prevent systemic HIV infection and allow time for a cellular immune response. Dendritic cells in the mucosa and skin are believed to be the initial target for HIV infection or capture.[6] In a primate model, simian immunodeficiency virus (SIV) remained localized in association with dendritic cells underlying the site of vaginal inoculation for the first 24 hours after exposure to cell-free virus.[7] Within 24 to 48 hours, these cells seemed to migrate to regional lymph nodes and present SIV to T lymphocytes. Cell-free and cell-associated SIV was detected in the peripheral blood within 5 days after inoculation.

Productive HIV infection occurs in a sequence of events involving initial capture and/or infection of dendritic target cells near the exposure site with subsequent transmission of HIV to susceptible T cells in regional lymph nodes. Each step in this sequence is a potential target for intervention. Early antiretroviral treatment plausibly prevents infection by blocking the infection of T cells, presumably in the regional lymph nodes. Interrupting or delaying the productive infection of T cells could also allow time for the development of specific cellular immunity directed against HIV in the exposed individual.

Animal studies provide evidence for an important role for the cellular immune system in HIV PEP. Intact cellular immunity was required for successful PEP in one mouse retroviral model.[8] Putkonen and coworkers[9] demonstrated robust specific cellular responses in macaques in which SIV infection was successfully prevented by PEP. These macaques developed a strong enough immune response that a second challenge with the same viral inoculum resulted in either no or significantly limited infection.

These data suggest that antiretroviral chemoprophylaxis administered soon after an exposure, in concert with cellular immunity, may prevent or inhibit systemic HIV infection. This preventive effect theoretically is caused by limiting proliferation of virus in dendritic cells in skin or in T cells in regional lymph nodes during the time in which the virus remains relatively localized. This effect may be bolstered by a robust cellular immune response.

Animal Models of Postexposure Prophylaxis

In general, PEP is most likely to be effective in animal models where the exposure inoculum is relatively low, when treatment is started soon after exposure (usually within 24 hours), and when treatment is continued for several days to weeks after inoculation.[10,11] In one study of SIV in macaques, all the animals receiving postexposure treatment for 28 days remained uninfected, only half the animals treated for 10 days remained uninfected, and none of the animals that received only 3 days of treatment were protected.[11] Similarly, delay in initiating prophylaxis was detrimental in this model. All of the animals that were treated within 24 hours of intravenous SIV infection remained uninfected, whereas only 50% of the animals that received treatment beginning 48 hours after infection and only 25% of the animals that received treatment beginning 72 hours after exposure were protected. Otten and colleagues[12] demonstrated similar findings in a macaque study assessing PEP after vaginal inoculation with HIV type 2. All animals treated within 48 hours were protected, whereas only some of the animals that received the antiretroviral agent 72 hours after inoculation remained uninfected.

Epidemiologic and Clinical Data Relevant to Occupational Postexposure Prophylaxis

Studies of prevention of mother-to-child transmission, including AIDS Clinical Trial Group protocol 076,[13] indicated a protective effect of zidovudine, which was attributable to a reduction in maternal HIV viral load (discussed by Cohn elsewhere in this issue).

In the CDC's retrospective case-control study of HCWs, zidovudine PEP was associated with an 81% reduction in the odds of infection after adjustment for relevant exposure risk factors.[4] This relatively small study was not designed to evaluate the merits of individual treatment regimens; thus, the effect of the drug regimen (dose, time to initiation, duration) on efficacy could not be determined. The study did not prove that treatment was effective, and limitations inherent in the design, including the small number of cases and the fact that cases and control subjects were not from the same cohort, must be considered.[14] Nevertheless, this study provided very suggestive epidemiologic evidence that zidovudine afforded some protection to exposed HCWs.

Antiretroviral chemoprophylaxis for occupational exposures to HIV has been in use in the United States since the late 1980s.[15] The numbers of occupational infections with HIV that have been reported to CDC have decreased steadily.[16] From 2000 to 2014, only a single case of occupational HIV infection was reported to CDC in 2010 (David Kuhar, CDC, personal communication, 2013). Most have been well-documented parenteral exposures (usually needlesticks from hollow-bore needles) to blood from a source patient known to be HIV-infected. Several factors have likely contributed to this decrease, including the use of primary exposure prevention strategies resulting in fewer exposures, the efficacy of highly active antiretroviral therapy in lowering the viral burden in HIV-infected source patients (both reducing the likelihood of their hospitalization and decreasing their need for, and numbers of, invasive procedures that place HCWs at risk for exposures), reduced reporting to CDC as the epidemic has matured and as staff have become knowledgeable about appropriate interventions, less aggressive case finding by the CDC and other local and state public health officials, and the use of PEP for occupational exposures.

Prophylaxis failures following occupational needlestick exposures have been documented in at least 24 instances.[17–20] In more than 75% of the instances of failure, zidovudine was used as a single agent. Only six instances of failure in the context of occupational needlestick exposure have been reported in association with the use of multiple-agent prophylaxis regimens.[19–23] In 15 of the 24 instances of PEP failure, the source patient for the exposure had previously been treated with one or more antiretroviral agents; thus, antiretroviral resistance possibly may, at least in part, explain the chemoprophylaxis failure. Additional factors may have contributed to these failures, including exposure to high HIV inocula, delayed initiation of prophylaxis, failure to achieve adequate drug concentrations, and inadequate treatment duration.

ASSESSMENT OF THE NEED FOR OCCUPATIONAL AND NONOCCUPATIONAL POSTEXPOSURE PROPHYLAXIS

Multiple factors should be considered when assessing an individual's need for PEP. First, prophylaxis should only be offered to individuals who are HIV-negative. Second, the type of exposure must be assessed, because per-event risk varies widely, depending on the exposure. Characteristics of the source patient are the final factors that need to be included in the initial risk assessment.

Baseline Human Immunodeficiency Virus Testing of Occupationally and Nonoccupationally Exposed Individuals

A negative result from an enzyme-linked immunosorbent assay for antibodies to HIV should be documented at the time of the initial assessment for occupational and nonoccupational exposures. If possible, HIV antibody testing should be done with a Food and Drug Administration (FDA)–approved rapid test kit with results available within 1 hour. HIV viral load testing may yield false-positive results if viral load levels below 1000 copies/uL are detected, and so is not recommended for baseline testing in the absence of signs or symptoms of acute retroviral syndrome. Fourth-generation HIV tests, which detect p24 antigen and conventional HIV antibodies, may be used in place of HIV antibody tests. Early antigen recognition with these assays reduces the window period for detection by approximately 5 days.

Testing of the Source Patient

In occupational settings, the source patient can often be quickly tested with a rapid HIV test. With the possible exception of the setting in which a high index of suspicion exists for acute infection (eg, source patient with risk factors and signs and symptoms consistent with acute retroviral syndrome), a negative HIV screening test obviates the need for PEP. Source patients should also be tested to assess hepatitis B and C virus serostatus, stage of disease, history of antiviral therapy, and viral load status for any and all of the bloodborne pathogens, if known. The source patient in nonoccupational exposures is rarely available for testing, so other epidemiologic factors must be considered. High-risk populations for which the toxicity and cost of PEP can be justified include men who have sex with men, men who have sex with both men and women, commercial sex workers, injection-drug users, persons with a history of incarceration, persons from a country where the seroprevalence of HIV is at least 1%, and persons who have a sexual partner belonging to one of these groups.

Exposure Type and Risk of Human Immunodeficiency Virus Transmission

Pooled data from multiple studies following HCWs with occupational HIV exposures suggest that the average risk of HIV transmission associated with percutaneous exposures to blood-contaminated sharp objects that have been used on HIV-infected individuals is approximately 0.32% (**Table 1**).[24] The estimated risk of mucocutaneous transmission is 0.03%. The risk of infection associated with intact skin exposure to HIV is too low to be detected in these studies.

Nonoccupational risk of HIV transmission depends on the nature of the exposure (see **Table 1**). The estimated risk of transmission following needle-sharing injection-drug use is higher than for any form of sexual exposure. The estimated risks associated with sexual exposures vary from 1.69% per act of male-to-female receptive anal intercourse[25] to 0.005% per act of insertive oral intercourse,[5] whereas only case reports have been received of female-to-female sexual transmission of HIV.[26] Per-act transmission probabilities are methodologically difficult to ascertain, because the time of seroconversion of the index case and the transmission to the partner, the number of unprotected sex acts, duration of exposure to HIV, and potential HIV cofactors at the time of transmission are rarely known precisely.[25] Exposures warranting PEP include unprotected sex, protected sex with condom failure, intravenous drug

Table 1	
Estimated per-act risk for acquisition of HIV, by exposure route	
Exposure Route	**Risk for 10,000 Exposures to an Infected Source**
Blood transfusion	9000
Needle-sharing injection-drug use	67
Receptive anal intercourse	50
Percutaneous needlestick	30
Receptive penile-vaginal intercourse	10
Insertive anal intercourse	65
Insertive penile-vaginal intercourse	5
Mucous membrane exposure (eg, splash)	3
Receptive oral intercourse	1
Insertive oral intercourse	0.5

Estimates of risk for transmission from sexual exposures assume no condom use.

Data from CDC. Antiretroviral postexposure prophylaxis after sexual, injection-drug use, or other nonoccupational exposure to HIV in the United States: recommendations from the U.S. Department of Health and Human Services. MMWR Recomm Rep 2004;54(RR-2):1–20.

use, or other mucosal or wound exposure. Exposures involving the insertive oral partner do not require PEP.

In general, chemoprophylaxis is recommended for exposures known to confer a transmission risk. Chemoprophylaxis should be considered for exposures with a "negligible risk." Chemoprophylaxis may not be warranted for exposures that do not pose a known transmission risk. In this framework, treatment is recommended for all percutaneous exposures to HIV and for mucosal and nonintact skin exposures, especially those that involve high titers of HIV (eg, blood from patients with advanced HIV disease, high viral load, or low $CD4^+$ counts). Treatment should be considered for small-volume, short-duration mucosal and nonintact skin exposure if the source patient is known or suspected to have a high circulating viral burden. In some institutions health care providers are give the option of electing prophylaxis for small-volume, short-duration mucosal and nonintact skin exposure. Although the associated risks for transmission are likely substantially smaller, some HCW prefer to take antiretroviral chemoprophylaxis to address even this smaller risk. Treatment is not indicated for most intact skin exposures. Occasionally a large-volume intact-skin exposure might warrant consideration for prophylaxis (eg, if a pheresis machine becomes disconnected with the pressure-pump engaged and the provider gets blood extensively on intact skin).

The actual risks associated with specific exposures to HIV are impossible to predict. Because the efficacy of PEP will likely never be demonstrated definitively in a clinical trial, and because the agents involved are associated with substantial toxic effects, PEP must be implemented with caution. Current US Public Health Service guidelines are based on exposures to blood or other potentially infectious materials known to contain HIV, not materials of uncertain HIV status.[27]

Decisions about treatment when the source material is not known to contain HIV should be based on a careful risk assessment, including a determination of (1) the probability of HIV infection in the source patient; (2) the type of exposure and the associated risk of HIV transmission with such an exposure, if HIV was, in fact, present; and (3) the risks associated with treatment for the exposed individual. In many "source unknown" exposures, the risk of transmission is negligible, and treatment is simply not indicated. Only if the assessment suggests that the risk of HIV transmission outweighs the risk of treatment is it reasonable to initiate the basic treatment regimen until test results or other data become available.

The use of antiretroviral chemoprophylaxis for nonoccupational exposures has been investigated extensively.[5,28–36] The rationale for providing PEP in these cases is no different from that for providing prophylaxis for occupational exposures. Clinicians should evaluate the circumstances of each exposure, provide counseling about the risks for infection and secondary transmission, and provide up-to-date information about the potential risks and benefits of antiretroviral chemotherapy. In many instances, the care provider's primary role is one of reassurance, inasmuch as the risk for transmission associated with many such community exposures may be small. Several reports describe instances where HIV transmission has been associated with human bites.[37,38] Evaluation of the bitten individual should include baseline testing for preexisting HIV infection, an offer of PEP if the patient is exposed to HIV, and follow-up identical to that described for other parenteral HIV exposures. Perpetrators of sexual assault are considered to be a high-risk population for HIV infection and PEP should be offered for these cases.[39–41]

DETAILS OF IMPLEMENTATION OF POSTEXPOSURE PROPHYLAXIS

This section discusses the factors that should be considered when choosing a treatment regimen, adverse effects associated with PEP, the timing and duration of PEP, and finally the follow-up needed for HIV exposures.

Choosing a Regimen for Postexposure Prophylaxis

Several factors influence the selection of antiretroviral drugs for prophylaxis regimen: (1) the type of exposure and the estimated risk of HIV transmission associated with the exposure, (2) the probability that drug-resistant virus strains are present in the source patient, (3) the safety profile and likelihood of the individual's adherence to the proposed treatment regimens, and (4) the cost of the agents.

CDC has recently published its fourth update of Public Health Guidelines for the Management of Occupational Exposures to HIV and Recommendations for Postexposure Prophylaxis.[27] Since publication of the previous update in 2005,[20] several novel antiretroviral agents have been granted FDA approval. In addition, investigators have amassed substantial experience regarding the safety and toxicity of these agents administered for prophylaxis for occupational and nonoccupational exposures. CDC and its expert consultants identified several challenges in the use and interpretation of the 2005 guidelines and addressed these issues in the 2013 recommendations.[27] Although no data demonstrate increased efficacy of three-drug HIV PEP regimens when compared with two-drug regimens, the 2013 guidelines recommend the routine administration of three agents for PEP and no longer recommend attempting to characterize the level of risk for HIV transmission for discrete exposures. CDC now recommends the combination of raltegravir, tenofovir, and emtricitabine as the "preferred" regimen for PEP, although not all experts agree. Some individuals emphasize the importance of the cost of these regimens and still favor a protease inhibitor as the third component of the regimen.[42] For alternative regimens, the 2013 guidelines recommend use of three agents (eg, two nucleoside reverse transcriptase inhibitors and either an integrase strand transfer inhibitor, a "ritonavir-boosted" protease inhibitor, or a nonnucleoside reverse transcriptase inhibitor [**Table 2**]). These alternative regimens may be indicated in unique clinical circumstances, but should be prescribed

Table 2
Recommended PEP for all occupational exposures to HIV

Preferred HIV PEP Regimen
  Raltegravir (Isentress), 400 mg PO twice daily
  Plus
  Tenofovir DF (Viread), 300 mg + emtricitabine (Emtriva), 200 mg (Truvada, 1 PO once daily)

Alternative Regimens (may combine one drug or drug pair from the left column with one pair of nucleoside/nucleotide reverse transcriptase inhibitors from the right column)

Raltegravir (Isentress)	Tenofovir DF (Viread) + emtricitabine (Emtriva); available as Truvada
Darunavir (Prezista) + ritonavir (Norvir)	Tenofovir DF (Viread) + lamivudine (Epivir)
Etravirine (Intelence)	Zidovudine (Retrovir) + lamivudine (Epivir); available as Combivir
Rilpivirine (Edurant)	Zidovudine (Retrovir) + emtricitabine (Emtriva)
Atazanavir (Reyataz) + ritonavir (Norvir)	
Lopinavir/ritonavir (Kaletra)	

Stribild (elvitegravir, cobicistat, tenofovir DF, emtricitabine), a complete fixed-dose combination regimen with no additional antiretrovirals needed

Alternative Antiretroviral Agents for Use as PEP ONLY with Expert Consultation
  Abacavir (Ziagen)
  Efavirenz (Sustiva)
  Enfuvirtide (Fuzeon)
  Fosamprenavir (Lexiva)
  Maraviroc (Selzentry)
  Saquinavir (Invirase)
  Stavudine (Zerit)
Antiretroviral Agents Generally Not Recommended for Use as PEP
  Didanosine (Videx EC)
  Nelfinavir (Viracept)
  Tipranavir (Aptivus)
Antiretroviral Agents Contraindicated as PEP
  Nevirapine (Viramune)

Data from Kuhar DT, Henderson DK, Struble KA, et al. Updated U.S. Public Health Service guidelines for the management of occupational exposures to HIV and recommendations for post-exposure prophylaxis. Infect Control Hosp Epidemiol 2013;34(9):875–92.

only after consultation with an expert experienced in the use of antiretrovirals and knowledgeable about the exposure.[27]

The 2013 CDC guidelines characterize three antiretroviral agents as "generally not recommended for use" in PEP (didanosine, nelfinavir, and tipranavir), and one agent, nevirapine, as "contraindicated" for use in prophylaxis. Nevirapine has been used extensively to treat HIV infection, but is known to have a greatly increased association with severe cutaneous and hepatic toxicity for males with CD4 counts greater than 400 cells/μL and females with CD4 counts greater than 250 cells/μL, counts that most persons who are candidates for PEP would be expected to have. Thus nevirapine is a poor choice for PEP and in fact is contraindicated.[43–47]

HIV resistance is an increasing concern, with resistance to all antiretroviral drugs reported and transmission of resistant strains.[48–52] Before treatment, 8% to 18% of HIV-infected persons have resistance to one or more antiretroviral drugs, and such resistance mutations adversely affect therapeutic response to the relevant drugs. If the source patient's resistance pattern for currently circulating virus is known, that information should guide selection of the PEP regimen. Drug resistance is most likely to be present among patients with high viral loads who are not responding to treatment or do not adhere to the treatment regimen. Unfortunately, if the resistance profile of the patient's virus has not been tested, clinical predictions about drug resistance are neither sensitive nor specific. Special genotypic and phenotypic tests to detect HIV resistance often are not readily available to provide immediate support for prophylactic treatment decisions. When drug resistance is suspected, PEP regimens should be based on the same principles used to select drugs for HIV-infected patients in whom treatment is failing. Many experts recommend a minimum of three agents that include the use of at least two drugs that the source patient has not taken in the recent past (ie, preceding 30 days). If the resistance is likely to involve an entire class of antiretroviral drugs (eg, protease inhibitors), including agents from other classes makes implicit sense.

Timing and Duration of Postexposure Prophylaxis

Treatment should be initiated as soon as possible after exposure. In most animal studies, efficacy is reduced when treatment is delayed for more than 24 hours.[11] Nonetheless, occupational and nonoccupational exposures to HIV should be regarded as urgent medical concerns. When indicated, chemoprophylaxis should be started as soon as practical (ie, within a few hours). When consultation is needed to select the best regimen, beginning the basic or expanded regimen until additional information is available may be the best course of action, rather than delaying the start of treatment. If local expertise is not available, additional resources for clinicians who need consultative assistance are listed in **Table 3**. The optimal duration of chemoprophylaxis is not known. A 4-week regimen is currently recommended.[27]

Adverse Effects of Postexposure Prophylaxis

Adverse effects have been associated with all agents and regimens used for PEP. The frequency, severity, duration, and reversibility of side effects are important considerations in formulating a prophylactic treatment regimen. Unusual or serious and

Table 3 Management of HIV exposure and PEP: HIV PEP resources and registries	
National HIV/AIDS Clinicians' Consultation Center: Postexposure Prophylaxis Hotline (PEPline)	Telephone: 888-448-4911 Web site: http://www.nccc.ucsf.edu/about_ nccc/pepline/
Antiretroviral Pregnancy Registry	Telephone (US and Canada): 800-258-4263 FAX: 800-800-1052 Telephone (International): 910-679-1598 Web site: http://www.apregistry.com Address: Research Park, 1011 Ashes Drive, Wilmington, NC 28405
US FDA MedWatch (for reporting unusual or severe toxicity to antiretroviral agents)	Telephone: 800-332-1088 Web site: www.fda.gov/medwatch/
CDC Cases of Public Health Importance (COPHI) coordinator (for reporting HIV infections in HCWs and failures of PEP)	Telephone: 404-639-2050

Data from Kuhar DT, Henderson DK, Struble KA, et al. Updated U.S. Public Health Service guidelines for the management of occupational exposures to HIV and recommendations for post-exposure prophylaxis. Infect Control Hosp Epidemiol 2013;34(9):875–92.

unexpected toxic effects of antiretroviral drugs should be reported to the manufacturer and the FDA (see **Table 3**). Although use of these drugs in the postexposure setting has become the standard of care, no agent has been approved or labeled for postexposure chemoprophylaxis for HIV exposures; therefore, all such use must be considered "off-label."

Much of the information about prophylactic treatment side effects was derived from studies of HCWs who took zidovudine alone, usually at doses higher than the currently recommended dose.[53] More than 50% of those treated reported at least one side effect, and about 30% stopped treatment because of symptoms. HCWs who took regimens that included two or more antiretroviral drugs experienced frequent side effects. In almost every instance, side effects ceased when treatment was stopped.

Side effects associated with HIV chemoprophylaxis are similar to (although strikingly more substantial than) those observed in HIV-infected patients, and most can be managed symptomatically (eg, acetaminophen for headache and myalgia, prochlorperazine for nausea, antimotility drugs for diarrhea). These adverse effects can decrease rates of adherence and completion of PEP regimens. Regular contact with the individual on PEP as frequently as possible is important to encourage course completion. Because these complications occur so commonly and because they can often be managed effectively with the symptomatic medications described previously, practitioners may wish to provide prescriptions for these agents with instructions, to "take this drug if you develop nausea, this one for diarrhea, etc."

Follow-up Assessments for Human Immunodeficiency Virus Postexposure Prophylaxis

In addition to baseline HIV testing, serologic testing for a documented HIV exposure is usually performed 6 weeks, 12 weeks, and 6 months after exposure.[27] Sequential testing is useful to allay fears; to document seronegativity; and, in rare instances, to diagnose HIV infection. Testing for more than 6 months is not routinely recommended, although individuals who become infected with hepatitis C virus after exposure to a source who is coinfected with HIV and hepatitis C virus should be tested again at 12 months.[27] Testing performed using fourth-generation combination antigen-antibody immunoassay permits earlier detection of HIV infection. The 2013 CDC guidelines indicate that, if fourth-generation HIV tests are used, HIV follow-up testing could be concluded at 4 months after the exposure.[27]

Symptoms of acute retroviral infection (eg, fever, lymphadenopathy, pharyngitis, rash, headache, profound fatigue) have been associated with approximately 80% of reported occupational infections, even when PEP was administered.[54] For this reason, all HIV-exposed persons should be advised to return for evaluation and HIV testing if an illness suggestive of the acute retroviral syndrome occurs. HIV antibody tests may be negative or indeterminate during early phases of the seroconversion illness. Immunoblot or viral load tests (quantitative HIV RNA polymerase chain reaction) may be more sensitive methods for detecting early infection should it be suspected, but are not indicated in the routine management of HIV exposures.

Individuals who elect to receive PEP after HIV exposure should return 48 to 72 hours after initiation of treatment for routine evaluation for signs and symptoms of drug toxicity and to make certain that all questions and concerns are addressed. The exposed patient should next be seen no later than 2 weeks after initiation of therapy and some practitioners prefer weekly evaluations for the first month. The clinician evaluating the patient should obtain a careful history, perform a focused physical examination, and obtain relevant laboratory tests appropriate to the drug regimen. As a general rule, a complete blood cell count and renal and hepatic chemical function tests are indicated. A random blood glucose measurement and a lipid profile should be considered whenever a protease inhibitor is included in the regimen.

Exposed individuals receiving PEP should be advised of the importance of completing the prescribed regimen. Many experts recommend use of barrier protection during sexual contact with partners and avoidance of shared blood-contaminated fomites (ie, razors and toothbrushes). Exposed individuals receiving PEP should be provided information about potential drug interactions and what medications not to take while taking the prophylactic drug regimen, the side effects of the drugs that have been prescribed and measures to minimize these effects, and methods of clinical monitoring for toxicity during the follow-up period. They should be alerted to the need for immediate evaluation of symptoms of the seroconversion illness and of symptoms suggestive of serious toxicity (eg, back or abdominal pain; pain on urination or blood in the urine; and symptoms of hyperglycemia, such as increased thirst or frequent urination).

REFERENCES

1. Prejean J, Song R, Hernandez A, et al. Estimated HIV incidence in the United States, 2006–2009. PLoS One 2011;6:e17502.
2. Joint United Nations Programme on HIV/AIDS (UNAIDS). Global report: UNAIDS report on the global AIDS epidemic 2013. Geneva (Switzerland): Joint United Nations Programme on HIV/AIDS (UNAIDS); 2013.
3. Centers for Disease Control and Prevention. Public Health Service statement on management of occupational exposure to human immunodeficiency virus, including considerations regarding zidovudine postexposure use. MMWR Recomm Rep 1990;39:1–14.
4. Cardo DM, Culver DH, Ciesielski CA, et al. A case-control study of HIV seroconversion in health care workers after percutaneous exposure. Centers for Disease Control and Prevention Needlestick Surveillance Group. N Engl J Med 1997;337:1485–90.
5. Centers for Disease Control and Prevention. Antiretroviral post-exposure prophylaxis after sexual, injection-drug use, or other non-occupational exposure to HIV in the United States. MMWR Recomm Rep 2005;54:1–20.
6. Blauvelt A. The role of skin dendritic cells in the initiation of human immunodeficiency virus infection. Am J Med 1997;102:16–20.
7. Spira AI, Marx PA, Patterson BK, et al. Cellular targets of infection and route of viral dissemination after an intravaginal inoculation of simian immunodeficiency virus into rhesus macaques. J Exp Med 1996;183:215–25.
8. Ruprecht RM, Bronson R. Chemoprevention of retroviral infection: success is determined by virus inoculum strength and cellular immunity. DNA Cell Biol 1994;13:59–66.
9. Putkonen P, Makitalo B, Bottiger D, et al. Protection of human immunodeficiency virus type 2-exposed seronegative macaques from mucosal simian immunodeficiency virus transmission. J Virol 1997;71:4981–4.
10. Black RJ. Animal studies of prophylaxis. Am J Med 1997;102:39–44.
11. Tsai CC, Emau P, Follis KE, et al. Effectiveness of postinoculation (R)-9-(2-phosphonylmethoxypropyl) adenine treatment for prevention of persistent simian immunodeficiency virus SIVmne infection depends critically on timing of initiation and duration of treatment. J Virol 1998;72:4265–73.
12. Otten RA, Smith DK, Adams DR, et al. Efficacy of postexposure prophylaxis after intravaginal exposure of pig-tailed macaques to a human-derived retrovirus (human immunodeficiency virus type 2). J Virol 2000;74:9771–5.

13. Connor EM, Sperling RS, Gelber R, et al. Reduction of maternal-infant transmission of human immunodeficiency virus type 1 with zidovudine treatment. Pediatric AIDS Clinical Trials Group Protocol 076 Study Group. N Engl J Med 1994; 331:1173–80.
14. Henderson DK. Postexposure treatment of HIV–taking some risks for safety's sake. N Engl J Med 1997;337:1542–3.
15. Henderson DK, Gerberding JL. Prophylactic zidovudine after occupational exposure to the human immunodeficiency virus: an interim analysis. J Infect Dis 1989;160:321–7.
16. Do AN, Ciesielski CA, Metler RP, et al. Occupationally acquired human immunodeficiency virus (HIV) infection: national case surveillance data during 20 years of the HIV epidemic in the United States. Infect Control Hosp Epidemiol 2003;24: 86–96.
17. Borba Brum MC, Dantas Filho FF, Yates ZB, et al. HIV seroconversion in a health care worker who underwent postexposure prophylaxis following needlestick injury. Am J Infect Control 2013;41:471–2.
18. Camacho-Ortiz A. Failure of HIV postexposure prophylaxis after a work-related needlestick injury. Infect Control Hosp Epidemiol 2012;33:646–7.
19. Centers for Disease Control and Prevention. Updated U.S. Public Health Service guidelines for the management of occupational exposures to HBV, HCV, and HIV and recommendations for postexposure prophylaxis. MMWR Recomm Rep 2001;50:1–52.
20. Panlilio AL, Cardo DM, Grohskopf LA, et al. Updated US. Public Health Service guidelines for the management of occupational exposures to HIV and recommendations for postexposure prophylaxis. MMWR Recomm Rep 2005;54:1–17.
21. Beltrami EM, Luo CC, de la Torre N, et al. Transmission of drug-resistant HIV after an occupational exposure despite postexposure prophylaxis with a combination drug regimen. Infect Control Hosp Epidemiol 2002;23:345–8.
22. Hawkins DA, Asboe D, Barlow K, et al. Seroconversion to HIV-1 following a needlestick injury despite combination post-exposure prophylaxis. J Infect 2001;43:12–5.
23. Perdue B, Wolderufael D, Mellors J, et al. HIV-1 transmission by a needle-stick injury despite rapid initiation of four-drug postexposure prophylaxis. Presented at the 6th Conference on retroviruses and opportunistic infections. Chicago, January 31–February 4, 1999.
24. Henderson DK. Human immunodeficiency virus in health care settings. In: Mandell GL, Bennett JE, Dolin R, editors. Principles and practice of infectious diseases. 7th edition. Philadelphia: Churchill Livingstone Elsevier; 2010. p. 3753–70.
25. Boily MC, Baggaley RF, Wang L, et al. Heterosexual risk of HIV-1 infection per sexual act: systematic review and meta-analysis of observational studies. Lancet Infect Dis 2009;9:118–29.
26. Centers for Disease Control and Prevention. Likely female-to-female sexual transmission of HIV—Texas, 2012. MMWR Morb Mortal Wkly Rep 2014;63: 209–12.
27. Kuhar DT, Henderson DK, Struble KA, et al. Updated US Public Health Service guidelines for the management of occupational exposures to human immunodeficiency virus and recommendations for postexposure prophylaxis. Infect Control Hosp Epidemiol 2013;34:875–92.
28. Barber TJ, Benn PD. Postexposure prophylaxis for HIV following sexual exposure. Curr Opin HIV AIDS 2010;5:322–6.
29. Bryant J, Baxter L, Hird S. Non-occupational postexposure prophylaxis for HIV: a systematic review. Health Technol Assess 2009;13:iii, ix–x, 1–60.

30. Crawford ND, Vlahov D. Progress in HIV reduction and prevention among injection and noninjection drug users. J Acquir Immune Defic Syndr 2010;55(Suppl 2): S84–7.
31. Ende AR, Hein L, Sottolano DL, et al. Nonoccupational postexposure prophylaxis for exposure to HIV in New York state emergency departments. AIDS Patient Care STDS 2008;22:797–802.
32. Fletcher JB, Rusow JA, Le H, et al. High-risk sexual behavior is associated with post-exposure prophylaxis non-adherence among men who have sex with men enrolled in a combination prevention intervention. J Sex Transm Dis 2013;2013: 210403.
33. Izulla P, McKinnon LR, Munyao J, et al. HIV postexposure prophylaxis in an urban population of female sex workers in Nairobi, Kenya. J Acquir Immune Defic Syndr 2013;62:220–5.
34. Poynten IM, Jin F, Mao L, et al. Nonoccupational postexposure prophylaxis, subsequent risk behaviour and HIV incidence in a cohort of Australian homosexual men. AIDS 2009;23:1119–26.
35. Puro V, De Carli G, Piselli P, et al. HIV incidence among men who have sex with men prescribed postexposure prophylaxis. AIDS 2012;26:1581–3 [author reply: 1583–4].
36. Roland ME. Postexposure prophylaxis after sexual exposure to HIV. Curr Opin Infect Dis 2007;20:39–46.
37. Lohiya GS, Tan-Figueroa L, Lohiya S. Human bites: bloodborne pathogen risk and postexposure follow-up algorithm. J Natl Med Assoc 2013;105:92–5.
38. Smoot EC, Choucino CM, Smoot MZ. Assessing risks of human immunodeficiency virus transmission by human bite injuries. Plast Reconstr Surg 2006; 117:2538–9.
39. Draughon JE, Anderson JC, Hansen BR, et al. Nonoccupational postexposure HIV prophylaxis in sexual assault programs: a survey of SANE and FNE program coordinators. J Assoc Nurses AIDS Care 2014;25:S90–100.
40. Draughon JE, Sheridan DJ. Nonoccupational postexposure prophylaxis following sexual assault in industrialized low-HIV-prevalence countries: a review. Psychol Health Med 2012;17:235–54.
41. Du Mont J, Myhr TL, Husson H, et al. HIV postexposure prophylaxis use among Ontario female adolescent sexual assault victims: a prospective analysis. Sex Transm Dis 2008;35:973–8.
42. Kuhar DT, Struble KA, Henderson DK. Reply to Tan, et al. Infect Control Hosp Epidemiol 2014;35:328–9.
43. Centers for Disease Control and Prevention. Serious adverse events attributed to nevirapine regimens for postexposure prophylaxis after HIV exposures– worldwide, 1997-2000. MMWR Morb Mortal Wkly Rep 2001;49:1153–6.
44. Johnson S, Baraboutis JG. Adverse effects associated with use of nevirapine in HIV postexposure prophylaxis for 2 health care workers. JAMA 2000;284:2722–3.
45. Patel SM, Johnson S, Belknap SM, et al. Serious adverse cutaneous and hepatic toxicities associated with nevirapine use by non-HIV-infected individuals. J Acquir Immune Defic Syndr 2004;35:120–5.
46. Rey D, L'Heritier A, Lang JM. Severe ototoxicity in a health care worker who received postexposure prophylaxis with stavudine, lamivudine, and nevirapine after occupational exposure to HIV. Clin Infect Dis 2002;34:418–9.
47. Sha BE, Proia LA, Kessler HA. Adverse effects associated with use of nevirapine in HIV postexposure prophylaxis for 2 health care workers. JAMA 2000;284: 2723.

48. Gagliardo C, Brozovich A, Birnbaum J, et al. A multicenter study of initiation of antiretroviral therapy and transmitted drug resistance in antiretroviral-naive adolescents and young adults with HIV in New York City. Clin Infect Dis 2014;58: 865–72.
49. Kleyn TJ, Liedtke MD, Harrison DL, et al. Incidence of transmitted antiretroviral drug resistance in treatment-naive HIV-1-infected persons in a large South Central United States clinic. Ann Pharmacother 2014;48(4):470–5.
50. Pennings PS. HIV drug resistance: problems and perspectives. Infect Dis Rep 2013;5:e5.
51. Snedecor SJ, Khachatryan A, Nedrow K, et al. The prevalence of transmitted resistance to first-generation non-nucleoside reverse transcriptase inhibitors and its potential economic impact in HIV-infected patients. PLoS One 2013;8: e72784.
52. Tilghman M, Perez-Santiago J, Osorio G, et al. Community HIV-1 drug resistance is associated with transmitted drug resistance. HIV Med 2014;15(6):339–46.
53. Lee LM, Henderson DK. Tolerability of postexposure antiretroviral prophylaxis for occupational exposures to HIV. Drug Saf 2001;24:587–97.
54. Ciesielski CA, Metler RP. Duration of time between exposure and seroconversion in healthcare workers with occupationally acquired infection with human immunodeficiency virus. Am J Med 1997;102:115–6.

Human Immunodeficiency Virus Vaccines

Paul Goepfert, MD[a],*, Anju Bansal, PhD[b]

KEYWORDS

- HIV vaccines • Neutralizing antibodies • Binding antibodies • T cells • Viral vector
- Protein boost • DNA prime

KEY POINTS

- The currently available clinical vaccines are based on inducing type-specific immunity, which is unlikely to work for a genetically diverse pathogen such as HIV.
- A recent HIV vaccine trial demonstrated 31% efficacy against HIV infection, but no protection against clinical markers of disease progression in those infected despite vaccination.
- The modest vaccine efficacy has led to the identification of new nonneutralizing (binding) antibodies that correlated with vaccine efficacy.
- Improvements to HIV-induced CD8 T-cell responses likely are needed if a vaccine is to change the clinical parameters of disease progression.
- Optimizing CD4 T-cell responses likely is essential to enhance the quality of antibodies and CD8 T cells.

INTRODUCTION

Despite tremendous advancements in the treatment of HIV-1 over the past 20 years, the number of new infections remains largely unchanged with an estimated 40,000 to 50,000 patients diagnosed annually with HIV infection in the United States[1] and over 2 million worldwide.[2] Up until recently, only behavioral modification modalities were effective in decreasing the number of new infections.[3] Fortunately, recent studies have demonstrated the effectiveness of male circumcision,[4–6] pre-exposure prophylaxis,[7–9] and treatment of infected partners[10] in significantly preventing HIV infection. Such improvements in therapeutic prevention modalities are likely to appreciably decrease the number of new HIV infections in the United States and globally. Nevertheless, based on the success of prior vaccines for many infectious diseases, an effective vaccine to prevent HIV infection and disease progression is thought to

[a] Division of Infectious Diseases, Department of Medicine, University of Alabama at Birmingham, 908, 20th Street South, CCB 328, Birmingham, AL 35294, USA; [b] Division of Infectious Diseases, Department of Medicine, University of Alabama at Birmingham, 845, 19th Street South, BBRB 557, Birmingham, AL 35294, USA
* Corresponding author.
E-mail address: paulg@uab.edu

Infect Dis Clin N Am 28 (2014) 615–631
http://dx.doi.org/10.1016/j.idc.2014.08.004
0891-5520/14/$ – see front matter © 2014 Elsevier Inc. All rights reserved.

id.theclinics.com

be the most effective potential weapon in controlling this global pandemic.[11–13] Many licensed vaccines elicit immune responses that confer T-cell-mediated and/or antibody-mediated protection from subsequent exposure.[14] Both arms of the adaptive immunity are needed in a vaccine, especially when dealing with highly variable pathogens. The immune mechanisms by which this antiviral effect is achieved are shown in **Fig. 1**. Therefore, it is thought that for an HIV vaccine to be highly efficacious, it must elicit robust humoral and cellular immune responses.[15]

Despite early optimism, the development of an effective HIV vaccine has been extremely difficult.[16,17] This cumbersome and lengthy process can take several years between transitioning from basic research to preclinical development to clinical trials. Furthermore, because HIV viral challenge is not possible, evaluation of vaccine efficacy in a high-risk group takes several additional years following the last vaccination. This evaluation is done to determine whether the vaccine recipients engaging in high-risk activities have decreased infection rates compared with placebos. To confound the timeline of vaccine development even further, gauging a vaccine's efficacy using validated immune assays can take additional time.

Several approaches have been tried to elicit humoral and/or cell-mediated immune responses. These approaches include using DNA and recombinant viral vectors to deliver HIV-1 gene products[18–20] as well as a protein boost using env-gp120.[21] Nevertheless, a large number of preclinical and clinical studies have been performed with largely disappointing results to date. Only 4 distinct vaccine regimens have made it

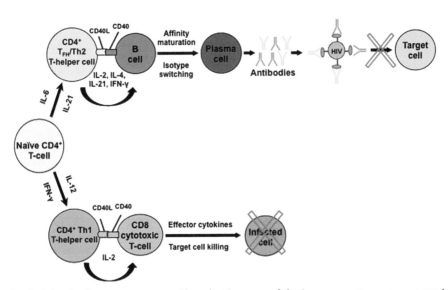

Fig. 1. Adaptive immune responses. The adaptive arms of the immune system are composed of the humoral (antibody) and the cellular (T-cell) -mediated immunity. (*top*) Naïve CD4+ T cells can differentiate into follicular helper CD4+ T cells (T$_{FH}$) or type 2 helper T cells (Th2) that are involved in B-cell activation following antigenic stimulation. Through the interaction of CD40 on B cells with CD40L on CD4 T cells, B cells will then differentiate into plasma cells, which will produce antibodies against HIV, thus preventing the virus from infecting target CD4 T cells. (*center*) Naïve CD4+ T cells differentiate into type 1 helper T cells (Th1) that can activate HIV-specific CD8+ T cells through the CD40/CD40L interaction. Activated CD8+ T cells mediate the killing of HIV-infected target T cells through the release of effector cytokines and molecules. (*bottom*) Naïve CD4+ T cells can differentiate into cytolytic CD4+ T cells, which can directly kill infected targets. IFN-γ, interferon-γ; IL, interleukin.

to clinical efficacy studies (**Fig. 2**),[21–25] and only 1 of these 4 studies has been somewhat successful in preventing infection or clinical markers of disease progression (**Fig. 3**).[25]

The first attempt included 2 clinical studies[26–28] that tested the efficacy of a bivalent monomer of the surface envelope glycoprotein (gp120). This design was tailored to induce type-specific antibody responses, a strategy that had worked for the hepatitis B vaccine.[29–31] Initially, the HIV vaccine approach was evaluated in healthy HIV-seronegative men and women at high risk of infection in the Americas and Europe. Despite successes seen in community engagement, rapid enrollment, safety, and follow-up, desirable efficacy with this product was not achieved.[23] A parallel study done in Thailand among intravenous drug users with a clade B/E env vaccine demonstrated similar findings.[21] Thus, although these 2 vaccines were safe, they did not elicit HIV-1-specific antibodies that effectively prevented infection. Because of the difficulties in generating antibodies that can bind and neutralize HIV virions, the focus of the HIV vaccinology field shifted toward generating T-cell responses.

The second vaccine regimen to be tested on a large scale consisted of a replication-defective adenovirus type 5 that encoded Gag, Pol, and Nef proteins. The inclusion of these immunogens that are not generally expressed on the surface of cells and lack Env in the vaccination regimen skewed the responses toward T cells, with the goal of preventing disease progression. This clinical trial was based on encouraging preclinical data in nonhuman primates, which showed that this vaccine induced potent

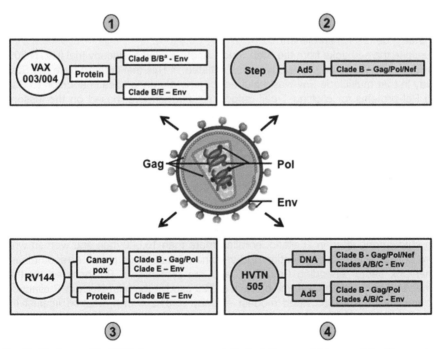

Fig. 2. Clade-specific HIV-1 immunogens and their delivery vehicles used in the vaccine regimens tested for efficacy. The HIV-1 clades from which the immunogens were derived, the type of immunogen used, and the mode of vaccine delivery are shown for each of the 4 vaccine regimens. At the center is a simplified depiction of an HIV virion showing the major proteins used as immunogens. [a] The bivalent clade B vaccine used in the VaxGen USA trial consisted of Env proteins from the MN and the GNE8 strains.

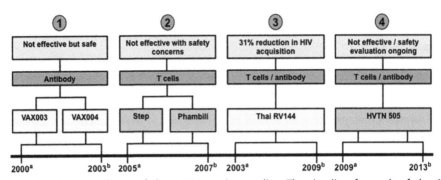

Fig. 3. Safety and efficacy of the 4 HIV vaccine studies. The timeline for each of the 4 vaccines is shown in terms of which year any given trial started[a] and ended[b]. The specific arms of the adaptive immunity measured are shown for each study. In addition, the safety and efficacy findings for each trial are summarized.

T-cell responses, which did not prevent infection but controlled infection and protected against progression to AIDS.[32] Nevertheless, clinical testing this vaccine strategy (the Step Study) failed to demonstrate protection against infection or clinical markers of disease progression in healthy men having sex with men (MSM).[22] In fact, safety concerns were raised when it appeared that a subset of vaccinees were at higher risk of infection.[33] The initial culprits for enhanced infection among vaccinees were thought to be high levels of pre-existing Ad5 antibody titers and/or lack of circumcision. Such concerns prompted stopping a sister study in South Africa (Phambili Study) before full enrollment.[34]

Despite the setbacks from the Step Study, another clinical efficacy trial (HVTN 505) that used rAD5 as a delivery vehicle was initiated.[35] This trial differed from the Step Study in that multiclade Env was included to generate antibodies in addition to Gag and Pol proteins for eliciting T-cell responses. Furthermore, based on the lessons learned from the Step Study, HVTN 505 enrolled Ad5-seronegative and circumcised MSM. Unfortunately, this study was also stopped before full follow-up because of a lack of efficacy in preventing infection or lowering viral loads in the infected vaccinees.[24] Fortunately, unlike the Step Study, there was no evidence of increased infection risk attributed to this vaccine.

The only vaccine study that has demonstrated some efficacy has been the RV144 Trial.[25] The move to go ahead with this study was fraught with controversy because its components were each shown to be nonefficacious[21,23] or poorly immunogenic by themselves,[36,37] prompting many skeptics to oppose this vaccine concept.[38] The study, conducted in Thailand, enrolled more than 16,000 men and women who were at increased risk of infection and vaccinated half of them with a recombinant canarypox vector encoding Env, Gag, and the protease of Pol boosted by this same vaccine combined with the bivalent gp120 used in the prior study in Thailand.[21] The vaccine regimen provided modest efficacy of 31.2% in protection against infection but no decrease in viral load set point in those who were infected despite vaccination.[25] Although the protection against infection just reached statistical significance, the findings were supported by a 60% efficacy 12 months following final vaccination, which subsequently waned. Follow-up analyses identified several immunologic correlates that were associated with the observed vaccine efficacy.[39,40] Although weak neutralizing antibodies were induced, binding antibodies of the immunoglobulin G (IgG) subtype to variable loops 1 and 2 of Env (V1V2) were found to be most predictive of vaccine efficacy.[41] Conversely, Env-specific plasma IgA antibodies targeting the C1 region directly correlated with infection rate. These IgA antibodies were not increasing the risk of infection but rather were diminishing the phagocytic enhancing effect of the V1/2-specific IgG antibodies.[42] Among vaccinees who became infected, sieving studies showed that the vaccine "selected" a signature mutation in the V2 loop, further supporting the importance of antibodies against this region.[43] Two recent studies have demonstrated that the IgG3 subtype was also associated with protection, suggesting that antibody-dependent cellular cytotoxicity (ADCC) may be playing an important role, because this antibody isotype is the best at engaging this process.[44,45] Interestingly, IgG3 responses were significantly lower in Vaxgen compared with the RV144 study.[44] The tremendous numbers of interrelated correlative findings support the validity of the partial efficacy seen in the RV144 Study.

Although the protection afforded in the RV144 study was modest, mathematical modeling studies have demonstrated that this vaccine regimen could be quite effective in reducing the number of new infections in select regions.[46,47] However, these assumptions are only valid if the vaccine regimen tested in RV144 truly prevents HIV infection. Therefore, confirmatory studies are planned using a similar vaccine regimen in both Thailand and Southern Africa. Furthermore, additional vaccine efficacy studies are planned in Southern Africa with other regimens that appear highly immunogenic in early clinical trials with the hopes of improving efficacy rates.

IMPROVEMENTS TO VACCINE-ELICITED IMMUNE RESPONSES
Antibodies

Antibodies able to directly neutralize virus are generally thought to be the best predictor of vaccine efficacy, and this immune response has correlated well with vaccine-induced protection for diseases such as polio, hepatitis B, and measles.[48] However, other effective vaccines largely induce nonneutralizing antibodies that are likely protecting through their functional attributes.[49] The latter likely occurs from antibodies able to bind to the pathogen via their variable domain. The Fc portion of the antibody-bound pathogen is then more efficiently recognized by immune cells through the Fc receptor. Depending on the type of the cell engaged, several processes are initiated, such as phagocytosis, complement-mediated cellular lysis, and ADCC, all resulting in pathogen clearance.[50–56] The latter function is especially interesting to the vaccine field going forward in light of the correlation with protection seen in the RV144 Study.[50] By modulating the vector, enveloping the antigen, and coadministering with a variety of adjuvants, numerous groups are hoping to enhance the functional antibody responses to improve the next generation of HIV vaccine regimens.

It was also intriguing that the vaccine regimen used in the RV144 Study provided up to 60% efficacy at 1 year following the final immunization, but this effectiveness rapidly declined in conjunction with antibody responses.[45,57–59] It is possible, therefore, that inducing a greater magnitude of antibody responses alone will significantly improve the observed vaccine efficacy. To this end, studies are underway to evaluate vaccine regimens designed to provide a better prime and enhanced boost to the immune response. This improvement will be evaluated with a combination of different adjuvants, vectors with enhanced delivery profiles, envelopes with better antigenic properties, and more frequent boosting, all in an attempt to increase the magnitude of the vaccine-induced antibody responses. Additional strategies to increase the durability of these responses also need to be explored.

Antibodies able to neutralize HIV by itself are rightfully understood to be the ideal vaccine-induced immune response.[60] Neutralizing antibodies are not only able to eliminate cell-free virus, they are also able to work in a coordinated fashion with other components of the immune system to combat infected cells. However, such anti-bodies have been extremely difficult to elicit with any HIV vaccine tested to date, inducing a response that is able to eliminate even a fraction of the easiest to neutralize viruses.[61] The reasons for these difficulties are many, including the vast diversity of HIV, whereby even antibodies able to neutralize a single viral clone are unable to do so for other highly related but genetically distinct viruses in the patient's quasispecies.[62,63] Such type-specific antibody immunity is not unusual and is in fact the predominant type of response that is seen for almost all commercially developed vaccines. For example, the human papilloma virus vaccine induces antibodies that are highly effective in protecting against the types of viruses included in the vaccine but can also cross-protect against ongogenic nonvaccine types that are not encoded by this immunogen.[64–66] Such a strategy works well when only a few viral subtypes cause significant disease (eg, 75% of cervical cancers are caused by HPV types 16 or 18); however, for HIV, virtually every functional virus is able to cause AIDS, and there are thousands of different HIV viral strains circulating in the human popu-lation.[67] If such viral diversity itself were not daunting enough, it is generally difficult to induce HIV neutralizing antibodies even with conventional vaccines. High-affinity antibodies generally require antibody maturation provided in large part by somatic mutations that evolve over time following exposure to the virus. For HIV, most potent neutralizing antibodies require extensive somatic hypermutation and are rarely induced before the first year following infection.[68–72] Many neutralizing antibody char-acteristics, such as a long CDR3 region, are also uncommon in humans and very diffi-cult to induce in mice, which are historically used as the preclinical model of vaccine development.[73]

Despite these difficulties, neutralizing antibodies are elicited in most HIV-infected individuals.[74,75] Furthermore, antibodies derived from a subset of individuals are able to neutralize a broad range of viruses.[68] In fact, over the past several years, a great number of potent, broadly neutralizing monoclonal antibodies have been devel-oped because of the development of novel technological advances.[76,77] Envelope antibodies were used as "baits" to identify B cells by flow cytometry, which are then sorted and examined genetically to reconstruct antibodies. These monoclonal anti-bodies are then screened for their ability to neutralize virus, and many have been found to have broad potency. The ability to solve the structure of envelope in combination with these broadly neutralizing antibodies has led to important insights into what may be needed to induce such responses with a vaccine.[78,79] Several groups are attempting to use "reverse vaccinology" to improve the antibody response.[80–82] This technique involves identifying a broadly neutralizing monoclonal antibody and then screening reactivity of this antibody against several envelope antigens.[83] Anti-gens with the highest reactivity would then be used as vaccines to determine whether they are able to induce the desired antibody response. This strategy may have to be combined with sequential vaccination, possibly with different forms of the envelope antigen to induce the antibody somatic hypermutation that appears to be required for generating broadly neutralizing antibody responses. Although these techniques are extremely complicated and not previously used in vaccine development, they are beginning to yield a set of blueprints from which it is hoped that more informed envelope antigen design can take place.

T Cells

It was understood early in HIV vaccine development that inducing antibodies of suf-ficient breadth to combat the diversity of HIV would be problematic.[84–86] Further-more, it was very difficult to induce antibodies that were able to neutralize primary

HIV isolates or those implicated in most acute infections. These concerns were enhanced with the findings that the AIDSVAX bivalent gp120 vaccine was unable to protect against infection in 2 separate trials.[21,23] At the same time, investigators noted that CD8 T-cell responses were able to kill HIV-infected cells with a much greater breadth than observed for antibodies.[87–91] CD8 T cells were also able to kill cells infected with primary HIV isolates. This renewed optimism led to the development of several vaccines whose primary goal was to induce T-cell responses. Preclinical data with these vaccine regimens looked very promising; however, protection against infection was generally not observed.[32,92,93] Rather, most of these vaccines protected against disease progression in vaccinated macaques and even this protection depended on the simian immunodeficiency virus (SIV) strain used for challenge.[94] Despite this optimism, 2 clinical studies have induced CD8 T-cell responses as the main response (Step Study) or in conjunction with antibody responses (HVTN 505), yet both studies failed to protect against infection or clinical markers of disease progression.[22,24] For the former study, eliciting CD8 T cells capable of preventing infection or impacting set-point viral load was one of the major endpoints.[22] Despite eliciting a high frequency and magnitude of response, this vaccine failed. One of the reasons for this is thought to be a narrow breadth of response.[95] Therefore, strategies that can enhance the breadth of CD8 T-cell responses are desirable for improving vaccine design. Despite the overall failure of this regimen, it is interesting to note that in vaccinees endowed with protective HLA-I alleles, Gag-specific responses correlated with a lower set point viral load.[96] The immune analyses for HVTN505 are ongoing.

Based on the above data, the field has serious doubts that a vaccine inducing CD8 T-cell responses as its primary immune response will ever be useful for an HIV vaccine; however, there is a wealth of information from both animal models and human data that these cells are essential for HIV viral control.[97–102] Even under the best of circumstances, antibodies are unlikely to protect against every infection and CD8 T cells will likely be needed for improved control following these infections. Furthermore, emerging data with what seems to be appropriate SIV challenge virus suggest that vaccine-induced CD8 T-cell responses are able to rapidly control infection to the extent that it is no longer detected in the challenged animals.[97,103–105] Although these data have used an unusual rhesus macaque cytomegalovirus vector, a more recent study was able to demonstrate protection against infection with a more conventional vectored approach that induced high levels of mucosal CD8 T-cell responses (David Masapoust, unpublished data, 2014). Such preclinical data point to an important role for CD8 T-cell responses to be included as part of a preventative vaccine in combination with reactive CD4 T cells and broadly reactive antibody responses, be it binding and/or neutralizing. As such, there is a renewed interest in developing vaccine regimens able to induce CD8 T-cell response of increased magnitude and breadth, especially those that are able to traffic to mucosal sites.

CD4 T-cell responses have received relatively little attention in terms of vaccine design, in part due to the fact the these cells are the primary targets of HIV infection and the arguable logic that enhancing these responses will inevitably fuel infection. However, there are preclinical data to suggest that HIV-specific CD4 T cells may be playing a contributing role in disease protection.[106] Furthermore, the RV144 correlates studies implicated CD4 T cells as playing at least a contributing role in protection against infection.[58] Although the exact mechanism behind this correlate of protection remains unknown, it is certainly plausible that CD4 T cells were enhancing the vaccine-induced antibody responses. In addition to its helper functions, CD4 T cells have long been known to possess lytic function; this characteristic was recently found to predict enhanced viral control when evaluated shortly after acute infection[107] and was also observed in RV144.[108] For these reasons, it seems prudent that future vaccine designs consider optimizing the induction and evaluation of CD4 T cells in addition to CD8 T cells.[109]

SUMMARY

HIV vaccine development began shortly after the discovery of this pathogen as the cause of AIDS.[110] Despite more than 25 years into the HIV epidemic, and the numerous preclinical and clinical testing of vaccines, only 4 regimens have reached efficacy stage testing to evaluate their ability to prevent HIV infection or disease progression. Only 1 of these 4 vaccine regimens was found to induce modest protection against infection but none demonstrated improved clinical markers of disease progression (lower set-point viral load and maintained CD4 T-cell counts) in those infected despite vaccination.[25] Nevertheless, a wealth of information was obtained from all of the efficacy trials, enhancing the understanding of the impact of vaccination on viral evolution and disease transmission.[111] For RV144, in particular, clear immune correlates of protection against HIV infection have been obtained; however, it is important to first confirm that the RV144 results are reproducible in subsequent trials in light of the modest rate of efficacy that just reached statistical significance. Fortunately, 2 studies are planned for near future (one in Thailand and one in Southern Africa), which will attempt to confirm the efficacy of the ALVAC/gp120 vaccine regimen.[112,113] These studies will determine whether the same correlates of HIV infection are seen as in the RV144 study, thereby potentially yielding valuable information to be used for more directed improvements in vaccine design.

It is important for the HIV vaccine field to continue to develop new products and move them rapidly to clinical testing.[111,114] Investigators should not be dissuaded by products that are significantly different than the RV144 regimen, as long as the scientific rationale is sound. This statement is especially pertinent in a field that has been fraught with focusing too heavily on a single vaccine platform without a developed backup plan when the former is found to be inefficacious. More importantly, a pertinent goal for the HIV vaccine field in the future is to increase the number of products tested concurrently for clinical efficacy. Sadly, this bar is not high enough, considering only 4 products have been tested for efficacy in more than 25 years of vaccine development. In general, vaccine development is an iterative process with more failures than successes, and significantly increasing the number of attempts is essential to developing a safe and effective HIV vaccine.

ACKNOWLEDGMENTS

We thank Victor Du for his help with the graphics.

REFERENCES

1. CDC. HIV incidence: centers for disease control. 2010. Available at: http://www.cdc.gov/hiv/statistics/surveillance/incidence/. Accessed May 6, 2014.
2. WHO. Global summary of the AIDS epidemic. World Health Organization; 2012 [cited May 6, 2014]. Available at: http://www.who.int/hiv/data/en/.
3. Vermund SH, Tique JA, Cassell HM, et al. Translation of biomedical prevention strategies for HIV: prospects and pitfalls. J Acquir Immune Defic Syndr

2013;63(Suppl 1):S12–25. http://dx.doi.org/10.1097/QAI.0b013e31829202a2. PubMed PMID: 23673881; PubMed Central PMCID: PMC3725750.

4. Auvert B, Taljaard D, Lagarde E, et al. Randomized, controlled intervention trial of male circumcision for reduction of HIV infection risk: the ANRS 1265 Trial. PLoS Med 2005;2(11):e298. http://dx.doi.org/10.1371/journal.pmed.0020298. PubMed PMID: 16231970; PubMed Central PMCID: PMC1262556.

5. Bailey RC, Moses S, Parker CB, et al. Male circumcision for HIV prevention in young men in Kisumu, Kenya: a randomised controlled trial. Lancet 2007; 369(9562):643–56. http://dx.doi.org/10.1016/S0140-6736(07)60312-2. PubMed PMID: 17321310.

6. Gray RH, Kigozi G, Serwadda D, et al. Male circumcision for HIV prevention in men in Rakai, Uganda: a randomised trial. Lancet 2007;369(9562):657–66. http://dx.doi.org/10.1016/S0140-6736(07)60313-4. PubMed PMID: 17321311.

7. Baeten JM, Donnell D, Ndase P, et al, Partners PrEP Study Team. Antiretroviral prophylaxis for HIV prevention in heterosexual men and women. N Engl J Med 2012;367(5):399–410. http://dx.doi.org/10.1056/NEJMoa1108524. PubMed PMID: 22784037; PubMed Central PMCID: PMC3770474.

8. Grant RM, Lama JR, Anderson PL, et al, iPrEx Study Team. Preexposure chemo-prophylaxis for HIV prevention in men who have sex with men. N Engl J Med 2010;363(27):2587–99. http://dx.doi.org/10.1056/NEJMoa1011205. PubMed PMID: 21091279; PubMed Central PMCID: PMC3079639.

9. Thigpen MC, Kebaabetswe PM, Paxton LA, et al, TDF2 Study Group. Antiretro-viral preexposure prophylaxis for heterosexual HIV transmission in Botswana. N Engl J Med 2012;367(5):423–34. http://dx.doi.org/10.1056/NEJMoa1110711. PubMed PMID: 22784038.

10. Cohen MS, Chen YQ, McCauley M, et al. Prevention of HIV-1 infection with early antiretroviral therapy. N Engl J Med 2011;365(6):493–505. http://dx.doi.org/10. 1056/NEJMoa1105243. PubMed PMID: 21767103; PubMed Central PMCID: PMC3200068.

11. Couch RB. Seasonal inactivated influenza virus vaccines. Vaccine 2008; 26(Suppl 4):D5–9. http://dx.doi.org/10.1016/j.vaccine.2008.05.076. PubMed PMID: 18602728; PubMed Central PMCID: PMC2643340.

12. Salk JE. Recent studies on immunization against poliomyelitis. Pediatrics 1953; 12(5):471–82. PubMed PMID: 13111847.

13. Salk JE. Principles of immunization as applied to poliomyelitis and influenza. Am J Public Health Nations Health 1953;43(11):1384–98. PubMed PMID: 13104698; PubMed Central PMCID: PMC1620430.

14. Kennedy RB, Ovsyannikova IG, Jacobson RM, et al. The immunology of smallpox vaccines. Curr Opin Immunol 2009;21(3):314–20. http://dx.doi.org/ 10.1016/j.coi.2009.04.004. PubMed PMID: 19524427; PubMed Central PMCID: PMC2826713.

15. Benmira S, Bhattacharya V, Schmid ML. An effective HIV vaccine: a combination of humoral and cellular immunity? Curr HIV Res 2010;8(6):441–9. PubMed PMID: 20636279.

16. Letvin NL. Progress and obstacles in the development of an AIDS vaccine. Nat Rev Immunol 2006;6(12):930–9. http://dx.doi.org/10.1038/nri1959. PubMed PMID: 17124514.

17. Kim JH, Rerks-Ngarm S, Excler JL, et al. HIV vaccines: lessons learned and the way forward. Curr Opin HIV AIDS 2010;5(5):428–34. http://dx.doi.org/10.1097/ COH.0b013e32833d17ac. PubMed PMID: 20978385; PubMed Central PMCID: PMC2990218.

18. Johnson JA, Barouch DH, Baden LR. Nonreplicating vectors in HIV vaccines. Curr Opin HIV AIDS 2013;8(5):412–20. http://dx.doi.org/10.1097/COH.0b013e 328363d3b7. PubMed PMID: 23925001.

19. Churchyard GJ, Morgan C, Adams E, et al, Network NHVT. A phase IIA randomized clinical trial of a multiclade HIV-1 DNA prime followed by a multiclade rAd5 HIV-1 vaccine boost in healthy adults (HVTN204). PLoS One 2011;6(8):e21225. http://dx.doi.org/10.1371/journal.pone.0021225. PubMed PMID: 21857901; PubMed Central PMCID: PMC3152265.

20. Goepfert PA, Horton H, McElrath MJ, et al, Network NHVT. High-dose recombinant Canarypox vaccine expressing HIV-1 protein, in seronegative human subjects. J Infect Dis 2005;192(7):1249–59. http://dx.doi.org/10.1086/432915. PubMed PMID: 16136469.

21. Pitisuttithum P, Gilbert P, Gurwith M, et al, Bangkok Vaccine Evaluation Group. Randomized, double-blind, placebo-controlled efficacy trial of a bivalent recombinant glycoprotein 120 HIV-1 vaccine among injection drug users in Bangkok, Thailand. J Infect Dis 2006;194(12):1661–71. http://dx.doi.org/10.1086/508748. PubMed PMID: 17109337.

22. Buchbinder SP, Mehrotra DV, Duerr A, et al, Step Study Protocol Team. Efficacy assessment of a cell-mediated immunity HIV-1 vaccine (the Step Study): a double-blind, randomised, placebo-controlled, test-of-concept trial. Lancet 2008;372(9653):1881–93. http://dx.doi.org/10.1016/S0140-6736(08)61591-3. PubMed PMID: 19012954; PubMed Central PMCID: PMC2721012.

23. Flynn NM, Forthal DN, Harro CD, et al, rgp HIV Vaccine Study Group. Placebo-controlled phase 3 trial of a recombinant glycoprotein 120 vaccine to prevent HIV-1 infection. J Infect Dis 2005;191(5):654–65. http://dx.doi.org/10.1086/ 428404. PubMed PMID: 15688278.

24. Hammer SM, Sobieszczyk ME, Janes H, et al. Efficacy trial of a DNA/rAd5 HIV-1 preventive vaccine. N Engl J Med 2013;369(22):2083–92. http://dx.doi.org/10. 1056/NEJMoa1310566. PubMed PMID: 24099601.

25. Rerks-Ngarm S, Pitisuttithum P, Nitayaphan S, et al, MOPH-TAVEG Investigators. Vaccination with ALVAC and AIDSVAX to prevent HIV-1 infection in Thailand. N Engl J Med 2009;361(23):2209–20. http://dx.doi.org/10.1056/ NEJMoa0908492. PubMed PMID: 19843557.

26. Billich A. AIDSVAX VaxGen. Curr Opin Investig Drugs 2004;5(2):214–21. PubMed PMID: 15043397.

27. Pitisuttithum P, Berman PW, Phonrat B, et al. Phase I/II study of a candidate vaccine designed against the B and E subtypes of HIV-1. J Acquir Immune Defic Syndr 2004;37(1):1160–5. PubMed PMID: 15319676.

28. Vanichseni S, Tappero JW, Pitisuttithum P, et al, Bangkok Vaccine Evaluation Group. Recruitment, screening and characteristics of injection drug users participating in the AIDSVAX B/E HIV vaccine trial, Bangkok, Thailand. AIDS 2004;18(2):311–6. PubMed PMID: 15075550.

29. Floreani A, Baldo V, Cristofoletti M, et al. Long-term persistence of anti-HBs after vaccination against HBV: an 18 year experience in health care workers. Vaccine 2004;22(5–6):607–10. PubMed PMID: 14741151.

30. Keating GM, Noble S. Recombinant hepatitis B vaccine (Engerix-B): a review of its immunogenicity and protective efficacy against hepatitis B. Drugs 2003; 63(10):1021–51. PubMed PMID: 12699402.

31. Poland GA, Jacobson RM. Clinical practice: prevention of hepatitis B with the hepatitis B vaccine. N Engl J Med 2004;351(27):2832–8. http://dx.doi.org/10. 1056/NEJMcp041507. PubMed PMID: 15625334.

32. Shiver JW, Fu TM, Chen L, et al. Replication-incompetent adenoviral vaccine vector elicits effective anti-immunodeficiency-virus immunity. Nature 2002;415(6869):331–5. http://dx.doi.org/10.1038/415331a. PubMed PMID: 11797011.
33. Duerr A, Huang Y, Buchbinder S, et al. Extended follow-up confirms early vaccine-enhanced risk of HIV acquisition and demonstrates waning effect over time among participants in a randomized trial of recombinant adenovirus HIV vaccine (Step Study). J Infect Dis 2012;206(2):258–66. http://dx.doi.org/10.1093/infdis/jis342. PubMed PMID: 22561365; PubMed Central PMCID: PMC3490694.
34. Volk JE, Hessol NA, Gray GE, et al. The HVTN503/Phambili HIV vaccine trial: a comparison of younger and older participants. Int J STD AIDS 2014;25(5):332–40. http://dx.doi.org/10.1177/0956462413506892. PubMed PMID: 24104693; PubMed Central PMCID: PMC3968181.
35. Catanzaro AT, Koup RA, Roederer M, et al, Vaccine Research Center 006 Study Team. Phase 1 safety and immunogenicity evaluation of a multiclade HIV-1 candidate vaccine delivered by a replication-defective recombinant adenovirus vector. J Infect Dis 2006;194(12):1638–49. http://dx.doi.org/10.1086/509258. PubMed PMID: 17109335; PubMed Central PMCID: PMC2428071.
36. Belshe RB, Stevens C, Gorse GJ, et al, National Institute of Allergy and Infectious Diseases AIDS Vaccine Evaluation Group and HIV Network for Prevention Trials(HIVNET). Safety and immunogenicity of a canarypox-vectored human immunodeficiency virus type 1 vaccine with or without gp120: a phase 2 study in higher- and lower-risk volunteers. J Infect Dis 2001;183(9):1343–52. http://dx.doi.org/10.1086/319863. PubMed PMID: 11294665.
37. Russell ND, Graham BS, Keefer MC, et al, National Institute of Allergy and Infectious Diseases HIV Vaccine Trials Network. Phase 2 study of an HIV-1 canarypox vaccine (vCP1452) alone and in combination with rgp120: negative results fail to trigger a phase 3 correlates trial. J Acquir Immune Defic Syndr 2007;44(2):203–12. http://dx.doi.org/10.1097/01.qai.0000248356.48501.ff. PubMed PMID: 17106277; PubMed Central PMCID: PMC2362395.
38. Burton DR, Desrosiers RC, Doms RW, et al. Public health. A sound rationale needed for phase III HIV-1 vaccine trials. Science 2004;303(5656):316. http://dx.doi.org/10.1126/science.1094620. PubMed PMID: 14726576.
39. Alam SM, Liao HX, Tomaras GD, et al. Antigenicity and immunogenicity of RV144 vaccine AIDSVAX clade E envelope immunogen is enhanced by a gp120 N-terminal deletion. J Virol 2013;87(3):1554–68. http://dx.doi.org/10.1128/JVI.00718-12. PubMed PMID: 23175357; PubMed Central PMCID: PMC3554162.
40. Robb ML, Rerks-Ngarm S, Nitayaphan S, et al. Risk behaviour and time as covariates for efficacy of the HIV vaccine regimen ALVAC-HIV (vCP1521) and AIDSVAX B/E: a post-hoc analysis of the Thai phase 3 efficacy trial RV 144. Lancet Infect Dis 2012;12(7):531–7. http://dx.doi.org/10.1016/S1473-3099(12)70088-9. PubMed PMID: 22652344; PubMed Central PMCID: PMC 3530398.
41. Zolla-Pazner S, deCamp A, Gilbert PB, et al. Vaccine-induced IgG antibodies to V1V2 regions of multiple HIV-1 subtypes correlate with decreased risk of HIV-1 infection. PLoS One 2014;9(2):e87572. http://dx.doi.org/10.1371/journal.pone.0087572. PubMed PMID: 24504509; PubMed Central PMCID: PMC3913641.
42. Tomaras GD, Ferrari G, Shen X, et al. Vaccine-induced plasma IgA specific for the C1 region of the HIV-1 envelope blocks binding and effector function

of IgG. Proc Natl Acad Sci U S A 2013;110(22):9019–24. http://dx.doi.org/10.1073/pnas.1301456110. PubMed PMID: 23661056; PubMed Central PMCID: PMC3670311.

43. Rolland M, Edlefsen PT, Larsen BB, et al. Increased HIV-1 vaccine efficacy against viruses with genetic signatures in Env V2. Nature 2012;490(7420):417–20. http://dx.doi.org/10.1038/nature11519. PubMed PMID: 22960785; PubMed Central PMCID: PMC3551291.

44. Chung AW, Ghebremichael M, Robinson H, et al. Polyfunctional Fc-effector profiles mediated by IgG subclass selection distinguish RV144 and VAX003 vaccines. Sci Transl Med 2014;6(228):228ra38. http://dx.doi.org/10.1126/scitranslmed.3007736. PubMed PMID: 24648341.

45. Yates NL, Liao HX, Fong Y, et al. Vaccine-induced Env V1-V2 IgG3 correlates with lower HIV-1 infection risk and declines soon after vaccination. Sci Transl Med 2014;6(228):228ra39. http://dx.doi.org/10.1126/scitranslmed.3007730. PubMed PMID: 24648342.

46. Hontelez JA, Nagelkerke N, Barnighausen T, et al. The potential impact of RV144-like vaccines in rural South Africa: a study using the STDSIM microsimulation model. Vaccine 2011;29(36):6100–6. http://dx.doi.org/10.1016/j.vaccine.2011.06.059. PubMed PMID: 21703321; PubMed Central PMCID: PMC3157643.

47. Nagelkerke NJ, Hontelez JA, de Vlas SJ. The potential impact of an HIV vaccine with limited protection on HIV incidence in Thailand: a modeling study. Vaccine 2011;29(36):6079–85. http://dx.doi.org/10.1016/j.vaccine.2011.06.048. PubMed PMID: 21718745.

48. Thakur A, Pedersen LE, Jungersen G. Immune markers and correlates of protection for vaccine induced immune responses. Vaccine 2012;30(33):4907–20. http://dx.doi.org/10.1016/j.vaccine.2012.05.049. PubMed PMID: 22658928.

49. Forthal D, Hope TJ, Alter G. New paradigms for functional HIV-specific non-neutralizing antibodies. Curr Opin HIV AIDS 2013;8(5):393–401. http://dx.doi.org/10.1097/COH.0b013e328363d486. PubMed PMID: 23924999.

50. Bonsignori M, Pollara J, Moody MA, et al. Antibody-dependent cellular cytotoxicity-mediating antibodies from an HIV-1 vaccine efficacy trial target multiple epitopes and preferentially use the VH1 gene family. J Virol 2012;86(21):11521–32. http://dx.doi.org/10.1128/JVI.01023-12. PubMed PMID: 22896626; PubMed Central PMCID: PMC3486290.

51. Chung AW, Navis M, Isitman G, et al. Activation of NK cells by ADCC antibodies and HIV disease progression. J Acquir Immune Defic Syndr 2011;58(2):127–31. http://dx.doi.org/10.1097/QAI.0b013e31822c62b9. PubMed PMID: 21792067; PubMed Central PMCID: PMC3175260.

52. Huber G, Banki Z, Lengauer S, et al. Emerging role for complement in HIV infection. Curr Opin HIV AIDS 2011;6(5):419–26. http://dx.doi.org/10.1097/COH.0b013e3283495a26. PubMed PMID: 21825871.

53. Isitman G, Stratov I, Kent SJ. Antibody-dependent cellular cytotoxicity and NK cell-driven immune escape in HIV infection: implications for HIV vaccine development. Adv Virol 2012;2012:637208. http://dx.doi.org/10.1155/2012/637208. PubMed PMID: 22611395; PubMed Central PMCID: PMC3350948.

54. Mazzolini J, Herit F, Bouchet J, et al. Inhibition of phagocytosis in HIV-1-infected macrophages relies on Nef-dependent alteration of focal delivery of recycling compartments. Blood 2010;115(21):4226–36. http://dx.doi.org/10.1182/blood-2009-12-259473. PubMed PMID: 20299515.

55. Torre D, Gennero L, Baccino FM, et al. Impaired macrophage phagocytosis of apoptotic neutrophils in patients with human immunodeficiency virus type 1

infection. Clin Diagn Lab Immunol 2002;9(5):983–6. PubMed PMID: 12204947; PubMed Central PMCID: PMC120074.

56. Wren L, Parsons MS, Isitman G, et al. Influence of cytokines on HIV-specific antibody-dependent cellular cytotoxicity activation profile of natural killer cells. PLoS One 2012;7(6):e38580. http://dx.doi.org/10.1371/journal.pone.0038580. PubMed PMID: 22701674; PubMed Central PMCID: PMC3372512.

57. Zolla-Pazner S, deCamp AC, Cardozo T, et al. Analysis of V2 antibody responses induced in vaccinees in the ALVAC/AIDSVAX HIV-1 vaccine efficacy trial. PLoS One 2013;8(1):e53629. http://dx.doi.org/10.1371/journal.pone.0053629. PubMed PMID: 23349725; PubMed Central PMCID: PMC3547933.

58. Haynes BF, Gilbert PB, McElrath MJ, et al. Immune-correlates analysis of an HIV-1 vaccine efficacy trial. N Engl J Med 2012;366(14):1275–86. http://dx.doi.org/10.1056/NEJMoa1113425. PubMed PMID: 22475592; PubMed Central PMCID: PMC3371689.

59. Montefiori DC, Karnasuta C, Huang Y, et al. Magnitude and breadth of the neutralizing antibody response in the RV144 and Vax003 HIV-1 vaccine efficacy trials. J Infect Dis 2012;206(3):431–41. http://dx.doi.org/10.1093/infdis/jis367. PubMed PMID: 22634875; PubMed Central PMCID: PMC3392187.

60. Mascola JR, Haynes BF. HIV-1 neutralizing antibodies: understanding nature's pathways. Immunol Rev 2013;254(1):225–44. http://dx.doi.org/10.1111/imr.12075. PubMed PMID: 23772623; PubMed Central PMCID: PMC3738265.

61. Montefiori DC, Mascola JR. Neutralizing antibodies against HIV-1: can we elicit them with vaccines and how much do we need? Curr Opin HIV AIDS 2009;4(5):347–51. http://dx.doi.org/10.1097/COH.0b013e32832f4a4d. PubMed PMID: 20048696; PubMed Central PMCID: PMC2879149.

62. Basu D, Kraft CS, Murphy MK, et al. HIV-1 subtype C superinfected individuals mount low autologous neutralizing antibody responses prior to intrasubtype superinfection. Retrovirology 2012;9:76. http://dx.doi.org/10.1186/1742-4690-9-76. PubMed PMID: 22995123; PubMed Central PMCID: PMC3477039.

63. Smith TL, van Rensburg EJ, Engelbrecht S. Neutralization of HIV-1 subtypes: implications for vaccine formulations. J Med Virol 1998;56(3):264–8. PubMed PMID: 9783696.

64. Toft L, Tolstrup M, Muller M, et al. Comparison of the immunogenicity of Cervarix and Gardasil human papillomavirus vaccines for oncogenic non-vaccine serotypes HPV-31, HPV-33, and HPV-45 in HIV-infected adults. Hum Vaccin Immunother 2014;10(5). PubMed PMID: 24553190.

65. Einstein MH, Baron M, Levin MJ, et al. Comparison of the immunogenicity and safety of Cervarix and Gardasil human papillomavirus (HPV) cervical cancer vaccines in healthy women aged 18-45 years. Hum Vaccin 2009;5(10):705–19. PubMed PMID: 19684472.

66. Einstein MH, Baron M, Levin MJ, et al. Comparison of the immunogenicity of the human papillomavirus (HPV)-16/18 vaccine and the HPV-6/11/16/18 vaccine for oncogenic non-vaccine types HPV-31 and HPV-45 in healthy women aged 18-45 years. Hum Vaccin 2011;7(12):1359–73. http://dx.doi.org/10.4161/hv.7.12.18282. PubMed PMID: 22048172; PubMed Central PMCID: PMC3338933.

67. Gaschen B, Taylor J, Yusim K, et al. Diversity considerations in HIV-1 vaccine selection. Science 2002;296(5577):2354–60. http://dx.doi.org/10.1126/science.1070441. PubMed PMID: 12089434.

68. Hraber P, Seaman MS, Bailer RT, et al. Prevalence of broadly neutralizing antibody responses during chronic HIV-1 infection. AIDS 2014;28(2):163–9. http://dx.doi.org/10.1097/QAD.0000000000000106. PubMed PMID: 24361678.

69. Klein F, Diskin R, Scheid JF, et al. Somatic mutations of the immunoglobulin framework are generally required for broad and potent HIV-1 neutralization. Cell 2013;153(1):126–38. http://dx.doi.org/10.1016/j.cell.2013.03.018. PubMed PMID: 23540694; PubMed Central PMCID: PMC3792590.

70. Medina-Ramirez M, Sanders RW, Klasse PJ. Targeting B-cell germlines and focusing affinity maturation: the next hurdles in HIV-1-vaccine development? Expert RevVaccines 2014;13(4):449–52. http://dx.doi.org/10.1586/14760584. 2014.894469. PubMed PMID: 24606603.

71. Doria-Rose NA, Schramm CA, Gorman J, et al. Developmental pathway for potent V1V2-directed HIV-neutralizing antibodies. Nature 2014. http://dx.doi. org/10.1038/nature13036. PubMed PMID: 24590074.

72. Liao HX, Lynch R, Zhou T, et al. Co-evolution of a broadly neutralizing HIV-1 antibody and founder virus. Nature 2013;496(7446):469–76. http://dx.doi.org/ 10.1038/nature12053. PubMed PMID: 23552890; PubMed Central PMCID: PMC3637846.

73. West AP Jr, Scharf L, Scheid JF, et al. Structural insights on the role of antibodies in HIV-1 vaccine and therapy. Cell 2014;156(4):633–48. http://dx.doi.org/10. 1016/j.cell.2014.01.052. PubMed PMID: 24529371.

74. Richman DD, Wrin T, Little SJ, et al. Rapid evolution of the neutralizing antibody response to HIV type 1 infection. Proc Natl Acad Sci U S A 2003;100(7):4144–9. http://dx.doi.org/10.1073/pnas.0630530100. PubMed PMID: 12644702; PubMed Central PMCID: PMC153062.

75. Wei X, Decker JM, Wang S, et al. Antibody neutralization and escape by HIV-1. Nature 2003;422(6929):307–12. http://dx.doi.org/10.1038/nature01470. PubMed PMID: 12646921.

76. Scheid JF, Mouquet H, Feldhahn N, et al. Broad diversity of neutralizing antibodies isolated from memory B cells in HIV-infected individuals. Nature 2009;458(7238): 636–40. http://dx.doi.org/10.1038/nature07930. PubMed PMID: 19287373.

77. Moody MA, Yates NL, Amos JD, et al. HIV-1 gp120 vaccine induces affinity maturation in both new and persistent antibody clonal lineages. J Virol 2012;86(14): 7496–507. http://dx.doi.org/10.1128/JVI.00426-12. PubMed PMID: 22553329; PubMed Central PMCID: PMC3416280.

78. Huang J, Ofek G, Laub L, et al. Broad and potent neutralization of HIV-1 by a gp41-specific human antibody. Nature 2012;491(7424):406–12. http://dx.doi. org/10.1038/nature11544. PubMed PMID: 23151583.

79. McLellan JS, Pancera M, Carrico C, et al. Structure of HIV-1 gp120 V1/V2 domain with broadly neutralizing antibody PG9. Nature 2011;480(7377):336–43. http://dx. doi.org/10.1038/nature10696. PubMed PMID: 22113616; PubMed Central PMCID: PMC3406929.

80. Burton DR, Ahmed R, Barouch DH, et al. A blueprint for HIV vaccine discovery. Cell Host Microbe 2012;12(4):396–407. http://dx.doi.org/10.1016/j.chom.2012. 09.008. PubMed PMID: 23084910; PubMed Central PMCID: PMC3513329.

81. Schief WR, Ban YE, Stamatatos L. Challenges for structure-based HIV vaccine design. Curr Opin HIV AIDS 2009;4(5):431–40. http://dx.doi.org/10.1097/COH. 0b013e32832e6184. PubMed PMID: 20048708.

82. Stamatatos LHIV. vaccine design: the neutralizing antibody conundrum. Curr Opin Immunol 2012;24(3):316–23. http://dx.doi.org/10.1016/j.coi.2012.04.006. PubMed PMID: 22595693.

83. Ahlers JD. All eyes on the next generation of HIV vaccines: strategies for inducing a broadly neutralizing antibody response. Discov Med 2014;17(94): 187–99. PubMed PMID: 24759623.

84. Daar ES, Li XL, Moudgil T, et al. High concentrations of recombinant soluble CD4 are required to neutralize primary human immunodeficiency virus type 1 isolates. Proc Natl Acad Sci U S A 1990;87(17):6574–8. PubMed PMID: 2395859; PubMed Central PMCID: PMC54579.

85. Golding H, D'Souza MP, Bradac J, et al. Neutralization of HIV-1. AIDS Res Hum Retroviruses 1994;10(6):633–43. PubMed PMID: 8074927.

86. Moore JP, Cao Y, Qing L, et al. Primary isolates of human immunodeficiency virus type 1 are relatively resistant to neutralization by monoclonal antibodies to gp120, and their neutralization is not predicted by studies with monomeric gp120. J Virol 1995;69(1):101–9. PubMed PMID: 7527081; PubMed Central PMCID: PMC188553.

87. Betts MR, Krowka J, Santamaria C, et al. Cross-clade human immunodeficiency virus (HIV)-specific cytotoxic T-lymphocyte responses in HIV-infected Zambians. J Virol 1997;71(11):8908–11. PubMed PMID: 9343257; PubMed Central PMCID: PMC192363.

88. Buseyne F, Chaix ML, Fleury B, et al. Cross-clade-specific cytotoxic T lymphocytes in HIV-1-infected children. Virology 1998;250(2):316–24. http://dx.doi.org/10.1006/viro.1998.9373. PubMed PMID: 9792842.

89. Ferrari G, Humphrey W, McElrath MJ, et al. Clade B-based HIV-1 vaccines elicit cross-clade cytotoxic T lymphocyte reactivities in uninfected volunteers. Proc Natl Acad Sci U S A 1997;94(4):1396–401. PubMed PMID: 9037064; PubMed Central PMCID: PMC19802.

90. McAdam S, Kaleebu P, Krausa P, et al. Cross-clade recognition of p55 by cytotoxic T lymphocytes in HIV-1 infection. AIDS 1998;12(6):571–9. PubMed PMID: 9583596.

91. Wilson SE, Pedersen SL, Kunich JC, et al. Cross-clade envelope glycoprotein 160-specific CD8+ cytotoxic T lymphocyte responses in early HIV type 1 clade B infection. AIDS Res Hum Retroviruses 1998;14(11):925–37. PubMed PMID: 9686639.

92. Amara RR, Villinger F, Altman JD, et al. Control of a mucosal challenge and prevention of AIDS by a multiprotein DNA/MVA vaccine. Science 2001; 292(5514):69–74. PubMed PMID: 11393868.

93. Barouch DH, Santra S, Schmitz JE, et al. Control of viremia and prevention of clinical AIDS in rhesus monkeys by cytokine-augmented DNA vaccination. Science 2000;290(5491):486–92. PubMed PMID: 11039923.

94. Friedrich TC, Watkins DI. The role of the SIV model in AIDS vaccine research. IAVI Rep 2005;9(2):1, 6–8. PubMed PMID: 16156073.

95. McElrath MJ, De Rosa SC, Moodie Z, et al. Step Study Protocol T. HIV-1 vaccine-induced immunity in the test-of-concept Step Study: a case-cohort analysis. Lancet 2008;372(9653):1894–905.   http://dx.doi.org/10.1016/S0140-6736(08)61592-5. PubMed PMID: 19012957; PubMed Central PMCID: PMC2774110.

96. Janes H, Friedrich DP, Krambrink A, et al. Vaccine-induced gag-specific T cells are associated with reduced viremia after HIV-1 infection. J Infect Dis 2013; 208(8):1231–9. http://dx.doi.org/10.1093/infdis/jit322. PubMed PMID: 23878319; PubMed Central PMCID: PMC3778967.

97. Hansen SG, Ford JC, Lewis MS, et al. Profound early control of highly pathogenic SIV by an effector memory T-cell vaccine. Nature 2011;473(7348):523–7. http://dx.doi.org/10.1038/nature10003. PubMed PMID: 21562493; PubMed Central PMCID: PMC3102768.

98. Kuroda MJ, Schmitz JE, Charini WA, et al. Emergence of CTL coincides with clearance of virus during primary simian immunodeficiency virus infection in

rhesus monkeys. J Immunol 1999;162(9):5127–33. PubMed PMID: 10227983.

99. Schmitz JE, Kuroda MJ, Santra S, et al. Control of viremia in simian immunodeficiency virus infection by CD8+ lymphocytes. Science 1999;283(5403):857–60. PubMed PMID: 9933172.

100. Perreau M, Levy Y, Pantaleo G. Immune response to HIV. Curr Opin HIV AIDS 2013;8(4):333–40. http://dx.doi.org/10.1097/COH.0b013e328361faf4. PubMed PMID: 23743723.

101. Jessen H, Allen TM, Streeck H. How a single patient influenced HIV research–15-year follow-up. N Engl J Med 2014;370(7):682–3. http://dx.doi.org/10.1056/NEJMc1308413. PubMed PMID: 24521131.

102. Shasha D, Walker BD. Lessons to be learned from natural control of HIV - future directions, therapeutic, and preventive implications. Front Immunol 2013;4:162. http://dx.doi.org/10.3389/fimmu.2013.00162. PubMed PMID: 23805139; PubMed Central PMCID: PMC3691556.

103. Hansen SG, Piatak M Jr, Ventura AB, et al. Immune clearance of highly pathogenic SIV infection. Nature 2013;502(7469):100–4. http://dx.doi.org/10.1038/nature12519. PubMed PMID: 24025770; PubMed Central PMCID: PMC3849456.

104. Hansen SG, Sacha JB, Hughes CM, et al. Cytomegalovirus vectors violate CD8+ T cell epitope recognition paradigms. Science 2013;340(6135):1237874. http://dx.doi.org/10.1126/science.1237874. PubMed PMID: 23704576; PubMed Central PMCID: PMC3816976.

105. Hansen SG, Vieville C, Whizin N, et al. Effector memory T cell responses are associated with protection of rhesus monkeys from mucosal simian immunodeficiency virus challenge. Nat Med 2009;15(3):293–9. http://dx.doi.org/10.1038/nm, 1935. PubMed PMID: 19219024; PubMed Central PMCID: PMC2720091.

106. Hel Z, Nacsa J, Tryniszewska E, et al. Containment of simian immunodeficiency virus infection in vaccinated macaques: correlation with the magnitude of virus-specific pre- and postchallenge CD4+ and CD8+ T cell responses. J Immunol 2002;169(9):4778–87 PubMed PMID: 12391187.

107. Soghoian DZ, Jessen H, Flanders M, et al. HIV-specific cytolytic CD4 T cell responses during acute HIV infection predict disease outcome. Sci Transl Med 2012;4(123):123ra25. http://dx.doi.org/10.1126/scitranslmed.3003165. PubMed PMID: 22378925; PubMed Central PMCID: PMC3918726.

108. de Souza MS, Ratto-Kim S, Chuenarom W, et al, Ministry of Public Health-Thai AVEGC. The Thai phase III trial (RV144) vaccine regimen induces T cell responses that preferentially target epitopes within the V2 region of HIV-1 envelope. J Immunol 2012;188(10):5166–76. http://dx.doi.org/10.4049/jimmunol.1102756. PubMed PMID: 22529301; PubMed Central PMCID: PMC3383859.

109. Streeck H, D'Souza MP, Littman DR, et al. Harnessing CD4(+) T cell responses in HIV vaccine development. Nat Med 2013;19(2):143–9. http://dx.doi.org/10.1038/nm. 3054. PubMed PMID: 23389614; PubMed Central PMCID: PMC3626561.

110. Zagury D, Bernard J, Cheynier R, et al. A group specific anamnestic immune reaction against HIV-1 induced by a candidate vaccine against AIDS. Nature 1988;332(6166):728–31. http://dx.doi.org/10.1038/332728a0. PubMed PMID: 3162762.

111. Bansal GP, Malaspina A, Flores J. Future paths for HIV vaccine research: Exploiting results from recent clinical trials and current scientific advances. Curr Opin Mol Ther 2010;12(1):39–46. PubMed PMID: 20140815.

112. Williamson AL, Rybiki E, Shephard E, et al. South African HIV-1 vaccine candidates - the journey from the bench to clinical trials. S Afr Med J 2012;102(6): 452–5. PubMed PMID: 22668934.

113. Vaccari M, Poonam P, Franchini G. Phase III HIV vaccine trial in Thailand: a step toward a protective vaccine for HIV. Expert Rev Vaccines 2010;9(9):997–1005. http://dx.doi.org/10.1586/erv.10.104. PubMed PMID: 20822342.

114. Cohen YZ, Dolin R. Novel HIV vaccine strategies: overview and perspective. Ther Adv Vaccines 2013;1(3):99–112. http://dx.doi.org/10.1177/2051013613494535. PubMed PMID: 24757518; PubMed Central PMCID: PMC3967667.

Finding a Cure for Human Immunodeficiency Virus-1 Infection

Joel N. Blankson, MD, PhD[a], Janet D. Siliciano, PhD[a],
Robert F. Siliciano, MD, PhD[a,b,*]

KEYWORDS

- HIV • Cure • Antiretroviral therapy • Retroviral persistence • Latent reservoir

KEY POINTS

- Human immunodeficiency virus (HIV)-1 can persist in a latent form that is not affected by immune responses or antiretroviral drugs.
- This latent reservoir is the major barrier to curing HIV-1 infection.
- Several recent developments have provided hope that a cure can be achieved, but many obstacles remain.

INTRODUCTION

Remarkable advances have been made in the treatment of human immunodeficiency virus (HIV)-1 infection, but in the entire history of the epidemic, only 1 patient seems to have been cured. Herein we review the fundamental mechanisms that render HIV-1 infection difficult to cure and then discuss recent clinical and experimental situations in which some form of cure has been achieved. Finally, we consider approaches that are currently being taken to develop a general cure for HIV-1 infection.

The Basic Biology of Retroviral Persistence

The idea that HIV-1 infection might be curable is bold. Fundamental aspects of the biology of HIV-1 make cure implausible. After HIV-1 enters a host cell, the viral genetic information is copied by the viral enzyme reverse transcriptase from RNA into a

This work was supported by the Martin Delaney CARE and DARE Collaboratories (National Institutes of Health grants AI096113 and 1U19AI096109), by an ARCHE Collaborative Research Grant from amfAR, the Foundation for AIDS Research (108165-50-RGRL), by the Johns Hopkins Center for AIDS Research (P30AI094189), by NIH grant 43222, and by the Howard Hughes Medical Institute.
[a] Department of Medicine, Johns Hopkins University School of Medicine, 733, North Broadway, Baltimore, MD 21205, USA; [b] Howard Hughes Medical Institute, 733, North Broadway, Baltimore, MD 21205, USA
* Corresponding author. Howard Hughes Medical Institute, 733, North Broadway, Baltimore, MD 21205.
E-mail address: rsiliciano@jhmi.edu

Infect Dis Clin N Am 28 (2014) 633–650
http://dx.doi.org/10.1016/j.idc.2014.08.007
0891-5520/14/$ – see front matter © 2014 Elsevier Inc. All rights reserved.

id.theclinics.com

double-stranded DNA molecule approximately 10,000 base pairs in length. This DNA copy is then inserted directly into the DNA of the host cell. The resulting proviral form of the viral genetic information persists in the host cell DNA, essentially functioning as a cellular gene, for as long as the cell survives. Although host cells have many interesting ways to defend themselves against retroviral infection,[1] they have no mechanism to eliminate the integrated viral genome (provirus). At the level of individual cells, infection is essentially permanent. The irreversible insertion of retroviral DNA into host cell chromosomes through the integration reaction confers upon the virus the stability of the host cells. Thus, a critical determinant of HIV-1 persistence is the lifespan of infected host cells. If the lifespan of an infected cell is short, and if de novo infection can be fully blocked, then cure is possible.

The lifespan of cells infected with HIV-1 was unknown until 1995 when 2 groups developed a way to analyze the turnover of free virus and infected cells in vivo in infected individuals.[2,3] In untreated patients, HIV-1 replicates continuously, even during the asymptomatic phase between acute infection and the development of AIDS.[4] Plasma virus levels are typically in the range of 10,000 to 100,000 copies of HIV-1 RNA per milliliter of plasma during this period. Over short times intervals (days to weeks), the levels of plasma virus remain roughly constant. George Shaw and David Ho realized that this is essentially a state of equilibrium in which the number of new cells becoming infected every day is roughly equal to the number of infected cells dying every day. If de novo infection is blocked with potent antiretroviral drugs, then the resulting decay in viremia should reflect the rate at which infected cells die. In landmark studies,[2,3] these investigators measured changes in plasma virus levels shortly after patients were started on a potent antiretroviral drug such as a nonnucleoside reverse transcriptase inhibitor or a protease inhibitor. They made the surprising discovery that plasma virus levels fall rapidly and dramatically when de novo infection is blocked. A key feature of all currently approved antiretroviral drugs is that they block de novo infection of susceptible cells. They do not affect virus production by cells that already have an integrated provirus. This is true even of the PIs, which do not block the release of virus particles, but instead prevent the maturation of the released particles into an infectious form.[5] The rapid decay in viremia observed when de novo infection is blocked indicates that the lifespan of the infected cells that produce most of the plasmas virus is very short. Currently, the half-life is estimated to be less than 1 day.[2,3,6]

It is unclear why most infected cells have a short half-life in vivo. It has been presumed that viral cytopathic effects lead to the death of cells that are expressing high levels of viral proteins, but the mechanisms remain unclear.[7] Interesting recent work suggests that the CD4[+] T-cell depletion characteristic of untreated HIV-1 infection may result from an inflammatory form of cells death termed pyroptosis, triggered by abortive infection of resting CD4[+] T cells.[7] However, this finding does not explain the rapid death of productively infected cells. Infected cells can also be lysed by virus-specific cytolytic T lymphocytes (CTL) if viral peptides are presented on the cell surface in association with major histocompatibility complex molecules.[8] Some retroviruses, like HIV-1, rapidly evolve escape mutations in epitopes recognized by CTL, thus thwarting this mechanism of elimination.[9] Studies in the simian immunodeficiency virus model of HIV-1 infection suggest that CTL do not actually shorten the half-life of infected cells in vivo, although they clearly have a role in controlling viral replication.[10,11] Although our understanding of the fate of infected cells in vivo is incomplete, the rapid decay of viremia in treated individuals makes it abundantly clear that most infected cells survive only a short period of time in the productively infected state.

Additional studies by Perelson and colleagues[12] of patients starting combination antiretroviral therapy (ART) detected a second phase in the viral decay curve that was due to a second population of infected cells with a somewhat longer half-life (about 2 weeks). The nature of this cell population was unknown at the time and remains unclear.[13] However, the finding that most of the plasma virus is produced by cells with a relatively short lifespan (days to weeks) raised the possibility that HIV-1 infection might be cured simply by blocking new infection events and waiting for previously infected cells to decay. In fact, analysis by Perelson and colleagues[12] suggested that cure could be achieved with 2 to 3 years of ART. These findings were the basis of much of the optimism about cure that accompanied the initial finding the ART could reduce viremia to below the limit of detection of clinical assays. Unfortunately, the hope that ART alone could produce a cure was not realized. At about the time that effective ART regimens were being introduced, a third population of infected cells with an extremely long half-life was identified[14,15] and shown to allow viral persistence in the fact of suppressive ART.[16-21] These cells are resting memory CD4+ T cells that harbor a latent form of the virus. They represent the primary barrier to a cure.

HUMAN IMMUNODEFICIENCY VIRUS-1 LATENCY

Viral latency is a reversibly nonproductive state of infection of individual cells. For some viruses, such as those of the herpes virus family, it is an important mechanism of persistence, allowing the virus to avoid immunologic clearance mechanisms between periods of active viral replication. Because HIV-1 replicates continuously in untreated individuals,[4] HIV-1 persistence does not seem to require latency. Rather, the virus evades host immune responses through the rapid evolution of variants that are not recognized by antibodies or CTL.[9,22,23] Thus, it was not necessarily expected that HIV-1 could establish a state of latent infection in vivo. HIV-1 latency seems to be a somewhat accidental consequence of its tropism for activated CD4+ T cells. The virus readily infects and replicates in CD4+ T cells that have become activated in response to some antigenic challenge. HIV-1 gene expression depends heavily on host transcription factors that are present in the nucleus of activated T cells, notably nuclear factor-κB and nuclear factor of activated T cell.[24,25] After antigen-drive activation, some CD4+ T cells transition back to a resting state as long-lived memory T cells capable of responding to the same antigen in the future. The resting state is largely nonpermissive for HIV-1 gene expression, in part because key host transcription factors are excluded from the nucleus in resting CD4+ T cells. The end result is a stably integrated but transcriptionally silent form of the virus in a long-lived memory T cell. This allows HIV-1 to persist simply as genetic information, 10^5 bases of DNA integrated somewhere into the 6×10^9 base pair diploid human genome. In this form, the virus can persist unaffected by immune responses or antiretroviral drugs. However, if the relevant memory T cell becomes activated again by a future encounter with antigen, it can resume virus production. In vivo evidence for this form of latent infection was first obtained in the mid 1990s with the demonstration that populations of resting CD4+ T cells from infected individuals contained cells with integrated HIV-1 DNA but did not produce virus unless the cells were activated.[14,15] A viral outgrowth assay in which resting CD4+ T cells are activated and cultured with CD4+ T cells from uninfected donors to allow outgrowth of virus was used to measure the frequency of latently infected cells.[16,26] The frequencies are extremely low, on the order of 1 per million resting CD4+ T cells. However, the frequencies do not decline even after prolonged period of treatment with ART,[16-21] and thus this latent reservoir is considered a major barrier to curing the infection (**Box 1**).[20,27] Intensive efforts are being directed at eliminating this reservoir to achieve a cure.[28]

DEFINING A CURE

Despite the renewed interest in HIV-1 eradication, it has become important to refine the definition of cure. Two types of cures are widely discussed.[29] In a sterilizing

---

Box 1
Key points regarding basic human immunodeficiency virus (HIV)-1 biology and the cure of HIV-1 infection

- Irreversible integration of the viral genome into host cell DNA confers on the virus the stability of the infected host cell.

- Most productively infected host cells die rapidly.

- Antiretroviral drugs act by blocking de novo infection of host cells and can produce a complete or near-complete inhibition of new infection events.

- Because productively infected cells die rapidly and ART blocks new infection, the infection would by curable with ART if there were no long-lived infected cell population.

- A long-lived population of resting memory CD4$^+$ T cells carrying latent, replication-competent HIV-1 genomes is present in all patients and represents a major barrier to curing the infection.

Abbreviation: ART, antiretroviral therapy.

---

cure, there is complete eradication of the virus. In light of the high fraction of defective viral genomes, this definition could be further refined as follows: A sterilizing cure eliminates all replication-competent forms of the virus so that no viral reservoirs remain. By this definition, a patient who retains some defective viral sequences would still be considered cured. Another form of cure is a functional cure in which the virus is not completely eradicated, but rather is held in check by the host immune system. A functional cure could be an intervention that renders patients with progressive disease able to permanently control viral replication to below the limit of detection, thereby preventing clinical immunodeficiency and transmission. Examples of both types of cure are discussed herein.

The first patient in whom a sterilizing cure seems to have been achieved is an HIV-1–infected adult male who was doing well on ART when he developed acute myelogenous leukemia.[30] This patient is widely known as the "Berlin patient," named after the site of his treatment. As part of the treatment for his leukemia, the Berlin patient underwent a bone marrow transplant from a carefully selected donor who was homozygous for a 32-base pair deletion in the HIV-1 coreceptor CCR5. ART was stopped at the time of the initial transplant, and despite a complex posttransplant course, the patient has remained aviremic off ART for longer than 5 years. Careful analysis of multiple samples from the patient with a variety of extremely sensitive techniques has failed to convincingly demonstrate persistence of HIV-1 in this patient,[31] and he is therefore considered to be the first patient to have been cured of an established HIV-1 infection. Interestingly, very different results were observed in 2 additional patients with HIV-1 infection who underwent bone marrow transplantation for other indications.[32] In these patients (known as the Boston patients), the donors were wild type for CCR5 and infection of susceptible donor cells was prevented by continuing ART throughout the transplant period. ART was stopped several years after transplantation, and the rebound in viremia, which normally occurs about 2 weeks after interruption of ART, was not observed. Instead, the patients maintained plasma virus levels below the limit of detection for many weeks, but both ultimately experienced a sudden and dramatic rebound of viremia to very high levels, 3 months and 8 months after ART interruption. In all 3 of these cases, the combination of the preparative regimens used and graft-versus-host disease eliminated most hematopoietic cells of host origin. Thus, the latent reservoir was reduced in a nonspecific fashion by targeting all host lymphoid cells. In the case of the Berlin patient, rebound did not occur because virus released from any residual latently infected cells would not be able to replicate in the HIV-1–resistant donor-derived cells that now comprise the patient's immune system. The viral rebounds observed in the Boston patients after prolonged periods of undetectable viremia nicely illustrate the concept of latent infection and suggest that only a very small number of residual, latently infected cells may be sufficient to rekindle the infection in the setting of a susceptible immune system.

The other widely discussed case of a sterilizing cure is that of the "Mississippi baby," an infant born to an infected mother who had no prenatal care.[33] At the time of birth, the baby's plasma HIV-1 RNA level was greater than 20,000 copies/mL, presumably reflecting in utero infection. An aggressive ART regimen was started within 31 hours of delivery and continued for 18 months. Treatment was then stopped against medical advice, but no rebound occurred for more than 1 year after interruption of ART. However, the baby was noted to have rebound viremia after an additional year of follow-up, similar to the Boston patients. In this situation, a potential cure was postulated because treatment was initiated before the latent reservoir in resting CD4$^+$ T cells was established. There are few memory T cells at birth, and the memory cell compartment is largely generated in response to encounter with antigen in postnatal life.[34] Yet, in the end, sterilizing cure was not achieved, probably because a small number of latently infected cells were generated before ART was started.

As noted, most productively infected cells have a very short half-life. The only HIV-1 reservoir that has been demonstrated to persist on a time scale of years in the setting of effective ART is the latent reservoir in resting CD4$^+$ T cells. In the absence of this reservoir, the infection would be curable if new infection of susceptible cells can be blocked. The Mississippi baby case is a testament to the remarkable efficacy of antiretroviral drugs.[35] Recent in vitro studies have provided evidence that the ability of ART regimens to block HIV-1 replication is actually much greater than previously thought.[35] Interestingly, hepatitis C virus does not establish a stable latent reservoir and is proving to be readily curable with direct acting antiviral drugs.[36,37] Together these findings emphasize the fact that the real barrier to HIV-1 cure is the latent reservoir. The Berlin patient seems to be the only example to date of a patient with an established latent reservoir who has been cured. Approaches to eliminate the latent reservoir are discussed at the end of this article.

IMMUNE CONTROL AND FUNCTIONAL CURE OF HUMAN IMMUNODEFICIENCY VIRUS-1 INFECTION

Given the difficulty of eliminating the latent reservoir, there has been great interest in another form of cure—the functional cure—in which the virus is not completely eradicated but rather is held in check by the host immune system. Elite controllers (EC) are patients who represent a model for a functional cure of HIV-1 infection.[38,39] These patients are seropositive for HIV-1, but maintain levels of HIV-1 RNA that are below the limit of detection of current clinical assays. They differ from long-term nonprogressors, who are defined as having stable CD4 counts and no clinical symptoms regardless of their HIV-1 RNA levels.[40] The mechanism of virologic control in EC has been the focus of intense research. Although several case reports have suggested that some EC and long-term nonprogressors are infected with attenuated or defective virus,[41,42] other studies have shown that replication-competent virus can be cultured from CD4$^+$ T cells in many EC.[43–45] Furthermore, full genome sequence analysis of replication-competent virus has not revealed any large deletions or signature mutations in the majority of EC,[43] and transmission pair studies have proven that some EC are infected with viruses that were sufficiently pathogenic to cause AIDS in the source patients.[46,47] Viral evolution has also been documented in EC,[48–50] and a recent study showed that isolates cultured from EC replicate vigorously in a humanized mouse model of HIV-1 infection, leading to profound depletion of human CD4+ T cells in these animals.[51] Taken together, the data suggest that unique host factors rather than infection with attenuated virus explain the majority of cases of elite control. Identification of these factors could clearly promote the development of strategies for a functional cure.

Among the many hypotheses to explain elite control, superior HIV-1–specific CD8+ T-cell activity is the best established correlate of immunity in these patients. Certain class I major histocompatibility complex alleles such as HLA-B*27 and HLA-B*57 are overrepresented in every cohort of ECs studied.[52–57] Furthermore, these HLA alleles are the only protective factors that have been identified in large, genome-wide association studies.[58,59] Class I HLA proteins present antigens to CD8+ T cells, and thus the mechanism by which these class I molecules contribute to protection from progressive HIV-1 infection may be through the presentation of critical HIV-1 epitopes to CD8+ T cells. The finding that HLA-B*27 and HLA-B*57 proteins present conserved immunodominant HIV-1 Gag epitopes is consistent with this hypothesis. Although the low fidelity of HIV-1 reverse transcriptase allows for the accumulation of mutations that can be quickly selected when pressure is applied, the fact that these targeted epitopes are in conserved regions of an essential viral protein means that the mutations will come at a significant fitness cost to the virus. In support of the T-cell hypothesis is the fact that HIV-1–specific CD8+ T cells in EC are more effective at producing multiple cytokines and chemokines and at killing HIV-1–infected CD4+ T cells than are CD8+ T cells from patients who have progressive disease.[60,61] Furthermore, in the nonhuman primate model of elite control, depletion of CD8+ T cells with antibody results in the transient loss of control of viral replication, which is reestablished when the effect of antibody levels decline and CD8+ T-cell numbers rebound.[62] However, not all patients who have these alleles become EC,[52] and a substantial number of EC do not have protective HLA alleles or strong CTL responses.[53,57] Thus, although protective class I HLA alleles and strong HIV-1–specific CTL responses clearly play a key role in many ECs, they cannot explain all aspects of elite control.

A functional cure of HIV-1 infection can sometimes be achieved in adults by the initiation of ART shortly after seroconversion. Early trials showed that after 1 year of treatment, some patients who began therapy during acute infection maintained low or undetectable plasma HIV-1 RNA levels when therapy was discontinued.[63] Unfortunately, this virologic control was short lived in the majority of patients, and by 3 years most of the patients were back on ART.[64] However, recent studies have documented the long-term control of viral replication in some patients who were treated during primary infection. Salgado and colleagues[65] described a patient who was treated during symptomatic primary infection and subsequently maintained plasma HIV-1 levels below the limit of detection for more than 9 years after stopping therapy. Saez-Cirion and colleagues[66] have described 14 patients who maintained some degree of control of viral replication after interrupting treatment. It is impossible to determine whether these patients were destined to become EC before treatment was initiated, but some patients had extremely high viral loads and severe clinical symptoms that are not often seen in primary infection in ECs.[66] Saez-Cirion and colleagues estimate that 5% to 15% of patients treated during acute HIV-1 infection may become posttreatment controllers. This is a much higher percentage than the reported prevalence of EC (0.5%–1 %) in many large cohorts.[40]

The mechanisms through which posttreatment controllers suppress viral replication are not known. It is unlikely that infection with attenuated virus can explain posttreatment control because many of these patients had high levels of viremia in primary infection. The frequency of HIV-1–infected cells in cohort studied by Saez-Cirion and colleagues[66] was much lower than the frequency normally seen in patients on highly active ART and seemed to be decreasing over time in some patients. However, in the case reported by Salgado and colleagues,[65] the frequency of HIV-1–infected cells was comparable to the frequency seen in patients on suppressive ART. Furthermore, in another trial in which patients were treated during acute HIV-1 infection, these patients were not able to control viral replication once treatment was discontinued, despite having very low frequencies of latently infected cells.[67] Thus, it seems that having a small HIV-1 reservoir is neither necessary nor sufficient for posttreatment control. Although early treatment leads to the maintenance of HIV-1–specific CD4+ T cells that are normally depleted during chronic HIV-1 infection, loss of control was shown to occur in the presence of these CD4+ T-cell responses, suggesting that they are not protective by themselves.[64] The posttreatment controllers studied by Saez-Cirion and colleagues[66] did not have a high incidence of the protective class I HLA alleles. Interestingly, HLA-B*35, an allele normally associated with rapid disease progression, was actually overrepresented in this cohort. Robust CD8+ T-cell responses that are often seen in EC were not found in these posttreatment controllers,[65,66] and in 1 case, high titers of neutralizing antibodies to autologous virus were excluded.[65] Thus, the mechanism of posttreatment control of HIV-1 replication remains elusive.

Elite control and posttreatment control are examples of a functional cure of HIV-1 infection, and understanding the mechanisms responsible for both phenomena may lead to the development of a therapeutic vaccine that controls HIV-1 replication without eradication (see the article by Goepfert and Bansal elsewhere in this issue). This may be analogous to the licensed vaccines for herpes zoster that significantly reduce the frequency of episodes of shingles but do not produce sterilizing immunity in older patients with chronic infection. It should be noted that, in some patients, elite control comes at a price. There is an higher incidence of immune activation[68,69] and higher levels of some inflammatory biomarkers in EC than patients on suppressive ART regimens.[70,71] Thus, the goal should be to develop a vaccine that prevents both viral replication and immune activation and inflammation.

TARGETING THE LATENT RESERVOIR

Although ART effectively suppresses viral replication, the basic biology of the latent reservoir necessitates lifelong treatment to avoid viral rebound.[20] In most patients, rebound occurs within about 2 weeks of treatment interruption.[72] There is genetic evidence that rebound originates from the latent reservoir,[73] although other stable reservoirs could certainly contribute. In any event, unless a method for inducing effective immune control of HIV-1 replication can be developed, elimination of the latent reservoir will be required before patients can be safely taken off ART. As discussed, allogeneic bone marrow transplantation with cells from a donor homozygous for a CCR5 deletion has generated the only cure of a patient with an established latent reservoir. However, the difficulties and dangers associated with bone marrow transplantation will likely restrict the use of this approach to patients who require transplantation for other conditions, and the current emphasis is on ways to directly target the latent reservoir.

The most widely discussed general approach for eliminating the reservoir, termed "shock and kill," involves the use of latency reversing agents to increase HIV-1 gene expression in latently infected cells. This would be done while the patients remained on ART so that the released virus would not infect new cells. It is hoped that the cells would then die from viral cytopathic effects or be lysed by virus-specific CTL. Recent studies of HIV-1–induced cell death focused on innate immune mechanisms that detect the presence of viral infection and initiate signaling cascades leading to cell death by pyroptosis.[7] However, innate immune sensors generally recognized viral DNA intermediates generated early in the virus life cycle, during the reverse transcription and integration reactions.[7,74] It is less clear that the innate immune system can sense the reactivation of a latent provirus, which essentially functions as a cellular gene. Thus, it is not yet clear that infected cells will die after the reversal of latency, particularly when latency is reversed using strategies that do not induce T-cell activation and high level virus gene expression. It may, therefore, be necessary to rely on other immune effector mechanisms, especially virus-specific CTL, to eliminate infected cells after reversal of latency. However, CTL responses wane in patients on ART, presumably owing the lack of antigen stimulation, and a recent in vitro study finds poor killing of infected cells after reversal of latency.[75] Thus, it may be necessary to combine some form of therapeutic vaccination with latency reversing strategies. Alternatively, novel immunotoxin-based strategies may promote the elimination of these cells.[76] In any event, the first step is to reverse latency and upregulate HIV-1 gene expression.

Early approaches to reversing latency relied on global T-cell activation.[77–79] However, there was often unacceptable toxicity, likely owing to the release of large amounts of proinflammatory cytokines by the activated T cells. These results focused discovery efforts on the identification of agents that reverse latency without global T-cell activation. The identification of latency reversing agents has been aided by a variety of in vitro models of HIV-1 latency, including transformed cell lines and primary $CD4^+$ T cells that have been infected with HIV-1 constructs carrying reporter genes and then manipulated in various ways to obtain cell populations in which viral gene expression has been turned off.[80–83] Using these in vitro models of latency, several different classes of latency reversing agents have been identified (reviewed by Xing and Siliciano[84]).

Most prominent among the classes of latency reversing agents identified to date are the histone deacetylase (HDAC) inhibitors. In in vitro models of HIV-1 latency, histones positioned at specific locations in the HIV-1 long terminal repeat can inhibit HIV-1 gene expression[85]; therefore, HDAC inhibitors, which have the effect of decreasing interactions between histones and DNA, might be expected to increase HIV-1 gene expression in the same way that they affect expression of a large number of host genes. Several HDAC inhibitors have been developed for the treatment of various cancers, and some of these drugs have been shown to reverse HIV-1 latency in model systems.[85–88] In a pioneering study, Archin and colleagues[89] showed that a single dose of the HDAC inhibitor vorinostat caused a modest increase in intracellular levels of transcripts containing HIV-1 *gag* sequences. However, a follow-up, multiple-dose study failed to show a sustained increase in HIV-1 gene expression.[90] Other studies with vorinostat have failed to detect induction of HIV-1 gene expression or virus production by cells from infected individuals.[91,92] In addition, there is some evidence that the effect of this drug on latent HIV-1 operates through a different mechanism.[93]

Another important class of latency of latency reversing agents are the protein kinase C agonists, including prostratin and bryostatin.[94–98] The activation of protein kinase C is a downstream event in the activation of T lymphocytes through the antigen receptor, and it is therefore not surprising that protein kinase C agonists induce expression of latent HIV-1 in several model systems. However, it is not yet clear whether these agents can be used safely in patients.

Several other classes of latency reversing agents have been identified, but in most cases the mechanisms involved have not yet been elucidated (reviewed by Xing and Siliciano[84]). A major problem is that the in vitro models used to study latency and to identify potential latency reversing agents may not accurately mimic the state of latently infected cells in vivo. A recent study[92] has shown that with the exception of bryostatin, the leading candidate latency reversing agents fail to upregulate HIV-1 gene expression in resting CD4$^+$ T cells from patients on ART. It is possible that no single agent may effectively convert the transcription environment in a resting T lymphocyte into one that is permissive for HIV-1 gene expression. Therefore, effective reversal of latency is likely to require carefully chosen combinations of agents.

ALTERNATIVE STRATEGIES

The "shock and kill" strategy is only one of many approaches currently being explored in the search for a cure (**Table 1**). As mentioned, early initiation of ART can reduce the size of the latent reservoir, but generally does not prevent its establishment. Near complete elimination of the reservoir has been achieved by allogeneic bone marrow transplantation strategies, but this dangerous intervention has only succeeded in a single case where the donor's cells were resistant to HIV-1 infection as a result of a homozygous deletion in CCR5. Recent advances in gene editing technology[99,100] will allow facile modification of host genes like CCR5 in hematopoietic stem cells, and several groups are exploring the idea of rendering hematopoietic stem cells from patients genetically resistant to HIV-1 infection for subsequent reinfusion into autologous hosts. The major problem with this strategy is how to eliminate all of the nonmodified host cells. In allogeneic transplantation, preparative regimens and graft-versus-host disease produce a near complete elimination of host cells, but this does not happen in autologous transplants. Ultimately, the most feasible general cure strategy may be one that enhances antiviral immune responses to the state that is observed in EC. Exciting recent studies by Hansen and colleagues[101] have shown that a cytomegalovirus-based simian immunodeficiency virus vaccine given before exposure can clear an established simian immunodeficiency virus infection, presumably by generating CTL that lyse infected cells before they have a chance to revert back to a latent state.

CLINICAL ASPECTS OF HUMAN IMMUNODEFICIENCY VIRUS-1 ERADICATION STRATEGIES

Although the cure case described has generated optimism regarding HIV-1 eradication, considerable challenges remain. One frequently voiced concern is that reversal of latency will lead to de novo infection of additional cells. Implicit in the "shock and kill" strategy is the possibility that virus production will transiently increase when latency reversing agents are administered. However, modern ART regimens have remarkable efficacy,[35] even in patients who begin therapy with very high levels of viremia. It is, therefore, likely that these regimens will prevent de novo infection by any viruses released after reversal of latency. As an additional safeguard, intensification of ART with additional antiretroviral drugs can be incorporated into latency reversing strategies.

Another important clinical question is how to measure the reservoir in clinical practice. At the present time, there is no clinical assay for the latent reservoir and no reason to measure it in the management of patients with HIV-1 infection. However, as clinical trials of eradication strategies proceed, it will become important to measure the reservoir. The reversal of latency in shock and kill trials may lead to transient

Table 1
Approaches to curing human immunodeficiency virus (HIV)-1 infection (see text for references)

Approach	Type of Cure	Example	Latent Reservoir	Population	Current Status
Shock and kill	Sterilizing	None yet	Must be reduced by >3 logs	Could be applied to all patients on ART	Effective latency reversing agents needed. Simultaneous boosting of CTL responses may be required. Long-term monitoring for rebound required.
Immune control of HIV replication	Functional	EC	Present but smaller than typical patient	Goal is to convert all patients to EC	Unclear how to render most patients able to control HIV replication.
Early treatment (adults)	Functional	Visconti cohort	Present	Limited to those treated very soon after exposure	Mechanism unclear, many studies in progress.
Early treatment (infants)	Sterilizing	Mississippi baby	Early treatment prevents formation	Infants born to infected mothers	Additional studies in progress.
Hematopoietic stem cell transplantation	Goal is a sterilizing cure	Berlin patient, Boston patients	Very small residual reservoir can lead to rebound unless donor cells are resistant	Currently, possible only in patients requiring bone marrow transplantation for other indications	One cure to date with resistant donor cells.

Abbreviations: ART, antiretroviral therapy; CTL, cytolytic T lymphocytes; EC, elite controllers.

increases in viremia detectable with standard clinical assays, which have a limit of detection of 20 to 50 copies of HIV-1 RNA/mL of plasma. Most patients on ART have trace levels of viremia that are below the limit of detection of standard clinical assays.[102–105] This residual viremia can be detected with special research assays and is typically on the order of 1 copy/mL of plasma. These assays may prove useful in eradication studies, but it is likely that an effective strategy will produce increases in viremia that are readily measureable, even with standard clinical assays.

Ultimately, it will be necessary to demonstrate that the intervention has reduced or eliminated the latent reservoir. The reservoir was originally defined with a quantitative viral outgrowth assay (QVOA) in which the frequency of resting CD4$^+$ T cells that produce replication-competent virus after cellular activation is determined.[15,16,26] This assay provides a definitive minimal estimate of the frequency of latently infected cells, but it is expensive and time consuming. Currently, the QVOA is performed only in a small number of research laboratories. Because of the low frequency of latently infected cells, this assay requires large volumes of blood (>100 mL) to detect latently infected cells. Any substantial (multi-log) reduction in the size of the reservoir would render the detection of latently infected cells unlikely without an even larger input of cells, for example, through leukapheresis.

It is also possible to detect the integrated viral genome with polymerase chain reaction (PCR) assays.[14,15,106–108] Interestingly, most PCR-based assays give infected cells frequencies that are 2 to 3 logs higher than, and poorly correlated with, infected cell frequencies determined by viral outgrowth.[109] An explanation for this discrepancy has recently been provided by Ho and colleagues.[110] They demonstrated that most viral genomes detected by PCR have readily identifiable defects that would preclude replication. These include lethal G→A hypermutation introduced by the host restriction factor APOBEC3G[1,111] and large internal deletions. However, this study also found that the number of intact genomes that were capable of giving rise to infectious virus significantly exceeded the number measured in the QVOA, suggesting that a single round of T-cell activation used in this assay does not induce all of the functional latent virus present. Thus, the QVOA likely underestimates the size of the reservoir, whereas PCR-based assays dramatically overestimate reservoir size.

Assuming that it will eventually be possible to develop strategies that produce a multi-log reduction in the latent reservoir, it is interesting to consider the clinical consequences for treated patients. With this degree of reduction, the latent reservoir may no longer be measurable with any assay. The only way to determine whether the strategy has been effective will be to interrupt ART and wait for viral rebound. Normally, rebound occurs within a few weeks of interruption. This time interval likely reflects the fact that multiple latently infected cells are being activated per day. The time to rebound represents the time needed for antiretroviral drug levels to decline sufficiently plus the time needed for viruses released from these cells to grow out. However, if the latent reservoir is reduced to the point where the activation rate is less than 1 cell per day, then there will be an additional, highly variable delay in time to rebound reflecting the stochastic activation of surviving cells in the reservoir. Some patients may experience a very late rebound, many months after interruption of ART. The Boston patients and the Mississippi baby described illustrate this problem. It is, therefore, important to consider how patients receiving eradication therapy will be monitored. Failure to detect and rapidly treat rebound viremia will likely result in reseeding of the latent reservoir to pre-intervention levels, and improper treatment or poor adherence could lead to the evolution of drug-resistant virus. Thus, curative strategies present many challenges beyond the initial step of finding ways to reverse HIV-1 latency.

SUMMARY

Given the remarkable success of ART and the likelihood that adherent patients on modern ART regimens will have a near normal lifespan,[112,113] it is important to consider how finding a cure for HIV-1 infection should fit into research priorities. The success of ART certainly alters the criteria for an acceptable curative protocol. No intervention that poses the risk of significant morbidity or mortality would be acceptable given the alternative of lifelong treatment with relatively well-tolerated ART regimens. Nevertheless, a strong justification for eradication research can be found in considering the global scale of the epidemic. A great deal of evidence suggests that all infected individuals should be treated with ART. Treatment outcomes are consistently better in patients who start treatment earlier.[114] The stability of the latent reservoir means that treatment should be continued for life.[19,20] The number of infected individuals stands at approximately 35 million and continues to increase. Whether it will be possible to treat this large and growing population with ART for life is unclear. Currently, well less than half of infected individuals are on ART, and many of them are receiving suboptimal regimens. A simple and safe eradication strategy that allows patients to stop ART for a significant period of time might allow treatment to be more widely distributed and thereby help to curb the spread of the epidemic.

REFERENCES

1. Sheehy AM, Gaddis NC, Choi JD, et al. Isolation of a human gene that inhibits HIV-1 infection and is suppressed by the viral VIF protein. Nature 2002;418: 646–50.
2. Ho DD, Neumann AU, Perelson AS, et al. Rapid turnover of plasma virions and CD4 lymphocytes in HIV-1 infection. Nature 1995;373:123–6.
3. Wei X, Ghosh SK, Taylor ME, et al. Viral dynamics in human immunodeficiency virus type 1 infection. Nature 1995;373:117–22.
4. Piatak M Jr, Saag MS, Yang LC, et al. High levels of HIV-1 in plasma during all stages of infection determined by competitive PCR. Science 1993;259:1749–54.
5. Rabi SA, Laird GM, Durand CM, et al. Multi-step inhibition explains HIV-1 protease inhibitor pharmacodynamics and resistance. J Clin Invest 2013;123:3848–60.
6. Perelson AS, Neumann AU, Markowitz M, et al. HIV-1 dynamics in vivo: Virion clearance rate, infected cell life-span, and viral generation time. Science 1996; 271:1582–6.
7. Doitsh G, Galloway NL, Geng X, et al. Cell death by pyroptosis drives CD4 T-cell depletion in HIV-1 infection. Nature 2014;505:509–14.
8. Walker BD, Chakrabarti S, Moss B, et al. HIV-specific cytotoxic T lymphocytes in seropositive individuals. Nature 1987;328:345–8.
9. Borrow P, Lewicki H, Wei X, et al. Antiviral pressure exerted by HIV-1-specific cytotoxic T lymphocytes (CTLs) during primary infection demonstrated by rapid selection of CTL escape virus. Nat Med 1997;3:205–11.
10. Wong JK, Strain MC, Porrata R, et al. In vivo CD8+ T-cell suppression of SIV viremia is not mediated by CTL clearance of productively infected cells. PLoS Pathog 2010;6:e1000748.
11. Klatt NR, Shudo E, Ortiz AM, et al. CD8+ lymphocytes control viral replication in SIVmac239-infected rhesus macaques without decreasing the lifespan of productively infected cells. PLoS Pathog 2010;6:e1000747.
12. Perelson AS, Essunger P, Cao Y, et al. Decay characteristics of HIV-1-infected compartments during combination therapy. Nature 1997;387:188–91.

13. Dinoso JB, Kim SY, Wiegand AM, et al. Treatment intensification does not reduce residual HIV-1 viremia in patients on highly active antiretroviral therapy. Proc Natl Acad Sci U S A 2009;106:9403–8.
14. Chun TW, Finzi D, Margolick J, et al. In vivo fate of HIV-1-infected T cells: quantitative analysis of the transition to stable latency. Nat Med 1995;1:1284–90.
15. Chun TW, Carruth L, Finzi D, et al. Quantification of latent tissue reservoirs and total body viral load in HIV-1 infection. Nature 1997;387:183–8.
16. Finzi D, Hermankova M, Pierson T, et al. Identification of a reservoir for HIV-1 in patients on highly active antiretroviral therapy. Science 1997;278:1295–300.
17. Wong JK, Hezareh M, Gunthard HF, et al. Recovery of replication-competent HIV despite prolonged suppression of plasma viremia. Science 1997;278:1291–5.
18. Chun TW, Stuyver L, Mizell SB, et al. Presence of an inducible HIV-1 latent reservoir during highly active antiretroviral therapy. Proc Natl Acad Sci U S A 1997;94: 13193–7.
19. Finzi D, Blankson J, Siliciano JD, et al. Latent infection of CD4+ T cells provides a mechanism for lifelong persistence of HIV-1, even in patients on effective combination therapy. Nat Med 1999;5:512–7.
20. Siliciano JD, Kajdas J, Finzi D, et al. Long-term follow-up studies confirm the stability of the latent reservoir for HIV-1 in resting CD4+ T cells. Nat Med 2003;9:727–8.
21. Strain MC, Gunthard HF, Havlir DV, et al. Heterogeneous clearance rates of long-lived lymphocytes infected with HIV: Intrinsic stability predicts lifelong persistence. Proc Natl Acad Sci U S A 2003;100:4819–24.
22. Richman DD, Wrin T, Little SJ, et al. Rapid evolution of the neutralizing antibody response to HIV type 1 infection. Proc Natl Acad Sci U S A 2003;100:4144–9.
23. Wei X, Decker JM, Wang S, et al. Antibody neutralization and escape by HIV-1. Nature 2003;422:307–12.
24. Nabel G, Baltimore D. An inducible transcription factor activates expression of human immunodeficiency virus in T cells. Nature 1987;326:711–3.
25. Bohnlein E, Lowenthal JW, Siekevitz M, et al. The same inducible nuclear proteins regulates mitogen activation of both the interleukin-2 receptor-alpha gene and type 1 HIV. Cell 1988;53:827–36.
26. Siliciano JD, Siliciano RF. Enhanced culture assay for detection and quantitation of latently infected, resting CD4+ T-cells carrying replication-competent virus in HIV-1-infected individuals. Methods Mol Biol 2005;304:3–15.
27. Richman DD, Margolis DM, Delaney M, et al. The challenge of finding a cure for HIV infection. Science 2009;323:1304–7.
28. The International AIDS Society Scientific Working Group on HIV Cure, Deeks SG, Autran B, et al. Towards an HIV cure: a global scientific strategy. Nat Rev Immunol 2012;12:607–14.
29. Dieffenbach CW, Fauci AS. Thirty years of HIV and AIDS: future challenges and opportunities. Ann Intern Med 2011;154:766–71.
30. Hutter G, Nowak D, Mossner M, et al. Long-term control of HIV by CCR5 Delta32/Delta32 stem-cell transplantation. N Engl J Med 2009;360:692–8.
31. Yukl SA, Boritz E, Busch M, et al. Challenges in detecting HIV persistence during potentially curative interventions: a study of the berlin patient. PLoS Pathog 2013;9:e1003347.
32. Henrich TJ, Hanhauser E, Sirignano MN, et al. HIV-1 rebound following allogeneic stem cell transplantation and treatment interruption. Ann Intern Med 2014;161:319–27.
33. Persaud D, Gay H, Ziemniak C, et al. Absence of detectable HIV-1 viremia after treatment cessation in an infant. N Engl J Med 2013;369:1828–35.

34. Farber DL, Yudanin NA, Restifo NP. Human memory T cells: generation, compartmentalization and homeostasis. Nat Rev Immunol 2014;14:24–35.

35. Jilek BL, Zarr M, Sampah ME, et al. A quantitative basis for antiretroviral therapy for HIV-1 infection. Nat Med 2012;18:446–51.

36. Ghany MG, Liang TJ. Current and future therapies for hepatitis C virus infection. N Engl J Med 2013;369:679–80.

37. Sulkowski MS, Gardiner DF, Rodriguez-Torres M, et al. Daclatasvir plus sofosbuvir for previously treated or untreated chronic HCV infection. N Engl J Med 2014; 370:211–21.

38. Blankson JN. Control of HIV-1 replication in elite suppressors. Discov Med 2010; 9:261–6.

39. Deeks SG, Walker BD. Human immunodeficiency virus controllers: mechanisms of durable virus control in the absence of antiretroviral therapy. Immunity 2007; 27:406–16.

40. Okulicz JF, Lambotte O. Epidemiology and clinical characteristics of elite controllers. Curr Opin HIV AIDS 2011;6:163–8.

41. Deacon NJ, Tsykin A, Solomon A, et al. Genomic structure of an attenuated quasi species of HIV-1 from a blood transfusion donor and recipients. Science 1995;270:988–91.

42. Alexander L, Weiskopf E, Greenough TC, et al. Unusual polymorphisms in human immunodeficiency virus type 1 associated with nonprogressive infection. J Virol 2000;74:4361–76.

43. Blankson JN, Bailey JR, Thayil S, et al. Isolation and characterization of replication-competent human immunodeficiency virus type 1 from a subset of elite suppressors. J Virol 2007;81:2508–18.

44. Lamine A, Caumont-Sarcos A, Chaix ML, et al. Replication-competent HIV strains infect HIV controllers despite undetectable viremia (ANRS EP36 study). AIDS 2007;21:1043–5.

45. Julg B, Pereyra F, Buzon MJ, et al. Infrequent recovery of HIV from but robust exogenous infection of activated CD4(+) T cells in HIV elite controllers. Clin Infect Dis 2010;51:233–8.

46. Bailey JR, O'Connell K, Yang HC, et al. Transmission of human immunodeficiency virus type 1 from a patient who developed AIDS to an elite suppressor. J Virol 2008;82:7395–410.

47. Buckheit RW 3rd, Allen TG, Alme A, et al. Host factors dictate control of viral replication in two HIV-1 controller/chronic progressor transmission pairs. Nat Commun 2012;3:716.

48. Bailey JR, Williams TM, Siliciano RF, et al. Maintenance of viral suppression in HIV-1-infected HLA-B*57+ elite suppressors despite CTL escape mutations. J Exp Med 2006;203:1357–69.

49. O'Connell KA, Brennan TP, Bailey JR, et al. Control of HIV-1 in elite suppressors despite ongoing replication and evolution in plasma virus. J Virol 2010;84: 7018–28.

50. Salgado M, Brennan TP, O'Connell KA, et al. Evolution of the HIV-1 nef gene in HLA-B*57 positive elite suppressors. Retrovirology 2010;7:94.

51. Salgado M, Swanson MD, Pohlmeyer CW, et al. HLA-B*57 elite suppressor and chronic progressor HIV-1 isolates replicate vigorously and cause CD4+ T cell depletion in humanized BLT mice. J Virol 2014;88:3340–52.

52. Migueles SA, Sabbaghian MS, Shupert WL, et al. HLA B*5701 is highly associated with restriction of virus replication in a subgroup of HIV-infected long term nonprogressors. Proc Natl Acad Sci U S A 2000;97:2709–14.

53. Pereyra F, Addo MM, Kaufmann DE, et al. Genetic and immunologic heterogeneity among persons who control HIV infection in the absence of therapy. J Infect Dis 2008;197:563–71.
54. Lambotte O, Boufassa F, Madec Y, et al. HIV controllers: a homogeneous group of HIV-1-infected patients with spontaneous control of viral replication. Clin Infect Dis 2005;41:1053–6.
55. Han Y, Lai J, Barditch-Crovo P, et al. The role of protective HCP5 and HLA-C associated polymorphisms in the control of HIV-1 replication in a subset of elite suppressors. AIDS 2008;22:541–4.
56. Sajadi MM, Constantine NT, Mann DL, et al. Epidemiologic characteristics and natural history of HIV-1 natural viral suppressors. J Acquir Immune Defic Syndr 2009;50:403–8.
57. Emu B, Sinclair E, Hatano H, et al. HLA class I-restricted T-cell responses may contribute to the control of human immunodeficiency virus infection, but such responses are not always necessary for long-term virus control. J Virol 2008;82:5398–407.
58. Fellay J, Shianna KV, Ge D, et al. A whole-genome association study of major determinants for host control of HIV-1. Science 2007;317:944–7.
59. International HIV Controllers Study, Pereyra F, Jia X, et al. The major genetic determinants of HIV-1 control affect HLA class I peptide presentation. Science 2010;330:1551–7.
60. Betts MR, Nason MC, West SM, et al. HIV nonprogressors preferentially maintain highly functional HIV-specific CD8+ T cells. Blood 2006;107:4781–9.
61. Migueles SA, Osborne CM, Royce C, et al. Lytic granule loading of CD8+ T cells is required for HIV-infected cell elimination associated with immune control. Immunity 2008;29:1009–21.
62. Friedrich TC, Valentine LE, Yant LJ, et al. Subdominant CD8+ T-cell responses are involved in durable control of AIDS virus replication. J Virol 2007;81:3465–76.
63. Rosenberg ES, Altfeld M, Poon SH, et al. Immune control of HIV-1 after early treatment of acute infection. Nature 2000;407:523–6.
64. Kaufmann DE, Lichterfeld M, Altfeld M, et al. Limited durability of viral control following treated acute HIV infection. PLoS Med 2004;1:e36.
65. Salgado M, Rabi SA, O'Connell KA, et al. Prolonged control of replication-competent dual- tropic human immunodeficiency virus-1 following cessation of highly active antiretroviral therapy. Retrovirology 2011;8:97. http://dx.doi.org/10.1186/1742-4690-8-97.
66. Saez-Cirion A, Bacchus C, Hocqueloux L, et al. Post-treatment HIV-1 controllers with a long-term virological remission after the interruption of early initiated antiretroviral therapy ANRS VISCONTI study. PLoS Pathog 2013;9:e1003211.
67. Chun TW, Justement JS, Murray D, et al. Rebound of plasma viremia following cessation of antiretroviral therapy despite profoundly low levels of HIV reservoir: Implications for eradication. AIDS 2010;24:2803–8.
68. Hunt PW, Brenchley J, Sinclair E, et al. Relationship between T cell activation and CD4+ T cell count in HIV-seropositive individuals with undetectable plasma HIV RNA levels in the absence of therapy. J Infect Dis 2008;197:126–33.
69. Andrade A, Bailey JR, Xu J, et al. CD4+ T cell depletion in an untreated HIV type 1-infected human leukocyte antigen-B*5801-positive patient with an undetectable viral load. Clin Infect Dis 2008;46:e78–82.
70. Krishnan S, Wilson EM, Sheikh V, et al. Evidence for innate immune system activation in HIV type 1-infected elite controllers. J Infect Dis 2014;209:931–9.

71. Noel N, Boufassa F, Lecuroux C, et al. Elevated IP10 levels are associated with immune activation and low CD4(+) T-cell counts in HIV controller patients. AIDS 2014;28:467–76.

72. Davey RT Jr, Bhat N, Yoder C, et al. HIV-1 and T cell dynamics after interruption of highly active antiretroviral therapy (HAART) in patients with a history of sustained viral suppression. Proc Natl Acad Sci U S A 1999;96:15109–14.

73. Joos B, Fischer M, Kuster H, et al. HIV rebounds from latently infected cells, rather than from continuing low-level replication. Proc Natl Acad Sci U S A 2008;105:16725–30.

74. Cooper A, Garcia M, Petrovas C, et al. HIV-1 causes CD4 cell death through DNA-dependent protein kinase during viral integration. Nature 2013;498:376–9.

75. Shan L, Deng K, Shroff NS, et al. Stimulation of HIV-1-specific cytolytic T lymphocytes facilitates elimination of latent viral reservoir after virus reactivation. Immunity 2012;36:491–501.

76. Denton PW, Long JM, Wietgrefe SW, et al. Targeted cytotoxic therapy kills persisting HIV infected cells during ART. PLoS Pathog 2014;10:e1003872.

77. Chun TW, Engel D, Mizell SB, et al. Effect of interleukin-2 on the pool of latently infected, resting CD4+ T cells in HIV-1-infected patients receiving highly active anti-retroviral therapy. Nat Med 1999;5:651–5.

78. Prins JM, Jurriaans S, van Praag RM, et al. Immuno-activation with anti-CD3 and recombinant human IL-2 in HIV-1-infected patients on potent antiretroviral therapy. AIDS 1999;13:2405–10.

79. Kulkosky J, Nunnari G, Otero M, et al. Intensification and stimulation therapy for human immunodeficiency virus type 1 reservoirs in infected persons receiving virally suppressive highly active antiretroviral therapy. J Infect Dis 2002;186:1403–11.

80. Jordan A, Bisgrove D, Verdin E. HIV reproducibly establishes a latent infection after acute infection of T cells in vitro. EMBO J 2003;22:1868–77.

81. Sahu GK, Lee K, Ji J, et al. A novel in vitro system to generate and study latently HIV-infected long-lived normal CD4+ T-lymphocytes. Virology 2006;355:127–37.

82. Burke B, Brown HJ, Marsden MD, et al. Primary cell model for activation-inducible human immunodeficiency virus. J Virol 2007;81:7424–34.

83. Spina CA, Anderson J, Archin NM, et al. An in-depth comparison of latent HIV-1 reactivation in multiple cell model systems and resting CD4+ T cells from aviremic patients. PLoS Pathog 2013;9:e1003834.

84. Xing S, Siliciano RF. Targeting HIV latency: Pharmacologic strategies toward eradication. Drug Discov Today 2013;18:541–51.

85. Van Lint C, Emiliani S, Ott M, et al. Transcriptional activation and chromatin remodeling of the HIV-1 promoter in response to histone acetylation. EMBO J 1996;15:1112–20.

86. He G, Ylisastigui L, Margolis DM. The regulation of HIV-1 gene expression: The emerging role of chromatin. DNA Cell Biol 2002;21:697–705.

87. Ylisastigui L, Archin NM, Lehrman G, et al. Coaxing HIV-1 from resting CD4 T cells: Histone deacetylase inhibition allows latent viral expression. AIDS 2004;18:1101–8.

88. Archin NM, Espeseth A, Parker D, et al. Expression of latent HIV induced by the potent HDAC inhibitor suberoylanilide hydroxamic acid. AIDS Res Hum Retroviruses 2009;25:207–12.

89. Archin NM, Liberty AL, Kashuba AD, et al. Administration of vorinostat disrupts HIV-1 latency in patients on antiretroviral therapy. Nature 2012;487:482–5.

90. Archin NM, Bateson R, Tripathy M, et al. HIV-1 expression within resting CD4 T-cells following multiple doses of vorinostat. J Infect Dis 2014;210:728–35.
91. Blazkova J, Chun TW, Belay BW, et al. Effect of histone deacetylase inhibitors on HIV production in latently infected, resting CD4(+) T cells from infected individuals receiving effective antiretroviral therapy. J Infect Dis 2012;206:765–9.
92. Bullen CK, Laird GM, Durand CM, et al. New ex vivo approaches distinguish effective and ineffective single agents for reversing HIV-1 latency in vivo. Nat Med 2014;20(4):425–9.
93. Contreras X, Schweneker M, Chen CS, et al. Suberoylanilide hydroxamic acid reactivates HIV from latently infected cells. J Biol Chem 2009;284:6782–9.
94. Kulkosky J, Culnan DM, Roman J, et al. Prostratin: activation of latent HIV-1 expression suggests a potential inductive adjuvant therapy for HAART. Blood 2001;98:3006–15.
95. Korin YD, Brooks DG, Brown S, et al. Effects of prostratin on T-cell activation and human immunodeficiency virus latency. J Virol 2002;76:8118–23.
96. Brooks DG, Hamer DH, Arlen PA, et al. Molecular characterization, reactivation, and depletion of latent HIV. Immunity 2003;19:413–23.
97. Williams SA, Chen LF, Kwon H, et al. Prostratin antagonizes HIV latency by activating NF-kappaB. J Biol Chem 2004;279:42008–17.
98. Beans EJ, Fournogerakis D, Gauntlett C, et al. Highly potent, synthetically accessible prostratin analogs induce latent HIV expression in vitro and ex vivo. Proc Natl Acad Sci U S A 2013;110:11698–703.
99. Didigu CA, Wilen CB, Wang J, et al. Simultaneous zinc-finger nuclease editing of the HIV coreceptors ccr5 and cxcr4 protects CD4+ T cells from HIV-1 infection. Blood 2014;123:61–9.
100. Ye L, Wang J, Beyer AI, et al. Seamless modification of wild-type induced pluripotent stem cells to the natural CCR5Delta32 mutation confers resistance to HIV infection. Proc Natl Acad Sci U S A 2014;111:9591–6.
101. Hansen SG, Piatak M Jr, Ventura AB, et al. Immune clearance of highly pathogenic SIV infection. Nature 2013;502:100–4.
102. Dornadula G, Zhang H, VanUitert B, et al. Residual HIV-1 RNA in blood plasma of patients taking suppressive highly active antiretroviral therapy. JAMA 1999;282:1627–32.
103. Palmer S, Wiegand AP, Maldarelli F, et al. New real-time reverse transcriptase-initiated PCR assay with single-copy sensitivity for human immunodeficiency virus type 1 RNA in plasma. J Clin Microbiol 2003;41:4531–6.
104. Maldarelli F, Palmer S, King MS, et al. ART suppresses plasma HIV-1 RNA to a stable set point predicted by pretherapy viremia. PLoS Pathog 2007;3:e46.
105. Palmer S, Maldarelli F, Wiegand A, et al. Low-level viremia persists for at least 7 years in patients on suppressive antiretroviral therapy. Proc Natl Acad Sci U S A 2008;105:3879–84.
106. O'Doherty U, Swiggard WJ, Jeyakumar D, et al. A sensitive, quantitative assay for human immunodeficiency virus type 1 integration. J Virol 2002;76:10942–50.
107. Yu JJ, Wu TL, Liszewski MK, et al. A more precise HIV integration assay designed to detect small differences finds lower levels of integrated DNA in HAART treated patients. Virology 2008;379:78–86.
108. Strain MC, Richman DD. New assays for monitoring residual HIV burden in effectively treated individuals. Curr Opin HIV AIDS 2013;8:106–10.
109. Eriksson S, Graf EH, Dahl V, et al. Comparative analysis of measures of viral reservoirs in HIV-1 eradication studies. PLoS Pathog 2013;9:e1003174.

110. Ho YC, Shan L, Hosmane NN, et al. Replication-competent noninduced proviruses in the latent reservoir increase barrier to HIV-1 cure. Cell 2013;155:540–51.
111. Harris RS, Bishop KN, Sheehy AM, et al. DNA deamination mediates innate immunity to retroviral infection. Cell 2003;113:803–9.
112. Nakagawa F, May M, Phillips A. Life expectancy living with HIV: Recent estimates and future implications. Curr Opin Infect Dis 2013;26:17–25.
113. Johnson LF, Mossong J, Dorrington RE, et al. Life expectancies of south African adults starting antiretroviral treatment: Collaborative analysis of cohort studies. PLoS Med 2013;10:e1001418.
114. Panel on Antiretroviral Guidelines for Adults and Adolescents. Guidelines for the use of antiretroviral agents in HIV-1-infected adults and adolescents. Department of Health and Human Services. 2013. Available at: http://Aidsinfo.nih.gov/contentfiles/lvguidelines/AdultandAdolescentGL.pdf.

Index

Note: Page numbers of article titles are in **boldface** type.

Infect Dis Clin N Am 28 (2014) 651–655
http://dx.doi.org/10.1016/S0891-5520(14)00073-7
0891-5520/14/$ – see front matter © 2014 Elsevier Inc. All rights reserved.

id.theclinics.com

United States Postal Service

Statement of Ownership, Management, and Circulation
(All Periodicals Publications Except Requestor Publications)

1. Publication Title	2. Publication Number	3. Filing Date
Infectious Disease Clinics of North America	0 0 1 - 5 5 6	9/14/14

4. Issue Frequency	5. Number of Issues Published Annually	6. Annual Subscription Price
Mar, Jun, Sep, Dec	4	$295.00

7. Complete Mailing Address of Known Office of Publication (Not printer) (Street, city, county, state, and ZIP+4®)

Elsevier Inc.
360 Park Avenue South
New York, NY 10010-1710

Contact Person
Stephen R. Bushing
Telephone (Include area code)
215-239-3688

8. Complete Mailing Address of Headquarters or General Business Office of Publisher (Not printer)

Elsevier Inc., 360 Park Avenue South, New York, NY 10010-1710

9. Full Names and Complete Mailing Addresses of Publisher, Editor, and Managing Editor (Do not leave blank)

Publisher (Name and complete mailing address)

Linda Belfus, Elsevier Inc., 1600 John F. Kennedy Blvd., Suite 1800, Philadelphia, PA 19103-2899

Editor (Name and complete mailing address)

Jessica McCool, Elsevier Inc., 1600 John F. Kennedy Blvd., Suite 1800, Philadelphia, PA 19103-2899

Managing Editor (Name and complete mailing address)

Adrianne Brigido, Elsevier Inc., 1600 John F. Kennedy Blvd., Suite 1800, Philadelphia, PA 19103-2899

10. Owner (Do not leave blank. If the publication is owned by a corporation, give the name and address of the corporation immediately followed by the names and addresses of all stockholders owning or holding 1 percent or more of the total amount of stock. If not owned by a corporation, give the names and addresses of the individual owners. If owned by a partnership or other unincorporated firm, give its name and address as well as those of each individual owner. If the publication is published by a nonprofit organization, give its name and address.)

Full Name	Complete Mailing Address
Wholly owned subsidiary of	1600 John F. Kennedy Blvd, Ste. 1800
Reed/Elsevier, US holdings	Philadelphia, PA 19103-2899

11. Known Bondholders, Mortgagees, and Other Security Holders Owning or Holding 1 Percent or More of Total Amount of Bonds, Mortgages, or Other Securities. If none, check box ☑ None

Full Name	Complete Mailing Address
N/A	

12. Tax Status (For completion by nonprofit organizations authorized to mail at nonprofit rates) (Check one)
The purpose, function, and nonprofit status of this organization and the exempt status for federal income tax purposes:
☑ Has Not Changed During Preceding 12 Months
☐ Has Changed During Preceding 12 Months (Publisher must submit explanation of change with this statement)

PS Form 3526, August 2012 (Page 1 of 3 (Instructions Page 3)) PSN 7530-01-000-9931 PRIVACY NOTICE: See our Privacy policy in www.usps.com

---

13. Publication Title	14. Issue Date for Circulation Data Below
Infectious Disease Clinics of North America	September 2014

15. Extent and Nature of Circulation			Average No. Copies Each Issue During Preceding 12 Months	No. Copies of Single Issue Published Nearest to Filing Date
a. Total Number of Copies (Net press run)			795	775
b. Paid Circulation (By Mail and Outside the Mail)	(1)	Mailed Outside-County Paid Subscriptions Stated on PS Form 3541. (Include paid distribution above nominal rate, advertiser's proof copies, and exchange copies)	495	472
	(2)	Mailed In-County Paid Subscriptions Stated on PS Form 3541 (Include paid distribution above nominal rate, advertiser's proof copies, and exchange copies)		
	(3)	Paid Distribution Outside the Mails Including Sales Through Dealers and Carriers, Street Vendors, Counter Sales, and Other Paid Distribution Outside USPS®	120	132
	(4)	Paid Distribution by Other Classes Mailed Through the USPS (e.g. First-Class Mail®)		
c. Total Paid Distribution (Sum of 15b (1), (2), (3), and (4))		▶	615	604
d. Free or Nominal Rate Distribution (By Mail and Outside the Mail)	(1)	Free or Nominal Rate Outside-County Copies Included on PS Form 3541	31	33
	(2)	Free or Nominal Rate In-County Copies Included on PS Form 3541		
	(3)	Free or Nominal Rate Copies Mailed at Other Classes Through the USPS (e.g. First-Class Mail)		
	(4)	Free or Nominal Rate Distribution Outside the Mail (Carriers or other means)		
e. Total Free or Nominal Rate Distribution (Sum of 15d (1), (2), (3) and (4))		▶	31	33
f. Total Distribution (Sum of 15c and 15e)		▶	646	637
g. Copies not Distributed (See instructions to publishers #4 (page #3))		▶	149	138
h. Total (Sum of 15f and g)		▶	795	775
i. Percent Paid (15c divided by 15f times 100)		▶	95.20%	94.82%

16. Total circulation includes electronic copies. Report circulation on PS Form 3526-X worksheet.

17. Publication of Statement of Ownership
If the publication is a general publication, publication of this statement is required. Will be printed in the December 2014 issue of this publication. ☐ Publication not required.

18. Signature and Title of Editor, Publisher, Business Manager, or Owner

Stephen R. Bushing – Inventory Distribution Coordinator

Date September 14, 2014

I certify that all information furnished on this form is true and complete. I understand that anyone who furnishes false or misleading information on this form or who omits material or information requested on the form may be subject to criminal sanctions (including fines and imprisonment) and/or civil sanctions (including civil penalties).

PS Form 3526, August 2012 (Page 2 of 3)

Moving?

Make sure your subscription moves with you!

To notify us of your new address, find your **Clinics Account Number** (located on your mailing label above your name), and contact customer service at:

Email: **journalscustomerservice-usa@elsevier.com**

800-654-2452 (subscribers in the U.S. & Canada)
314-447-8871 (subscribers outside of the U.S. & Canada)

Fax number: 314-447-8029

Elsevier Health Sciences Division
Subscription Customer Service
3251 Riverport Lane
Maryland Heights, MO 63043

*To ensure uninterrupted delivery of your subscription, please notify us at least 4 weeks in advance of move.

Printed and bound by CPI Group (UK) Ltd, Croydon, CR0 4YY

03/10/2024

01040485-0011